Name ______________________ Class ______________ Date ____

Skills Worksheet

Directed Reading

AF769476

Section: Body Organization

In the space provided, write which of the four basic kinds of tissue—*epithelial, nervous, connective,* or *muscle*—matches the term or phrase.

______________ **1.** blood

______________ **2.** enables movement of body structures

______________ **3.** cells that line body surfaces

______________ **4.** cells that carry information throughout the body

______________ **5.** bone

Read each question, and write your answer in the space provided.

6. Distinguish between smooth muscle and skeletal muscle.

____

____

7. What are embryonic stem cells?

____

____

8. Distinguish between tissues and organs.

____

____

9. What are the four body cavities, and what function do they each serve?

____

____

____

____

10. What four body functions help maintain homeostasis?

____

____

Name ______________________ Class ______________ Date ____________

Skills Worksheet

Directed Reading

Section: Skeletal System

In the space provided, explain how the terms in each pair differ in meaning.

1. axial skeleton, appendicular skeleton

____

____

____

2. bone marrow, periosteum

____

____

____

Read each question, and write your answer in the space provided.

3. What are Haversian canals?

____

____

____

4. What causes osteoporosis?

____

____

____

In the space provided, explain how the terms in each pair are related to each other.

5. joints, ligaments

____

____

____

6. immovable joints, slightly movable joints

____

____

In the space provided, write the letter of the description that best matches the term or phrase.

______	**7.** saddle joint	**a.** joint found in the shoulders and hips
______	**8.** pivot joint	**b.** joint found at the base of the thumbs
______	**9.** ball and socket joint	**c.** joint found at the top of the spine

Name ______________________ Class ______________ Date ____________

Skills Worksheet

Directed Reading

Section: Muscular System

Complete each statement by writing the correct term or phrase in the space provided.

1. Muscles can move body parts because muscles are attached to

______________________ .

2. Dense bands of connective tissue, called ______________________ , attach skeletal muscles to bones.

3. A(n) ______________________ muscle causes a joint to bend.

4. A(n) ______________________ muscle causes a joint to straighten.

Read each question, and write your answer in the space provided.

5. What are three important characteristics of muscle tissue?

____

____

____

6. Distinguish between myofibrils and sarcomeres.

____

____

____

In the space provided, write the letter of the description that best matches the term or phrase.

______ **7.** actin

______ **8.** ATP

______ **9.** aerobic energy pathway

______ **10.** myosin

______ **11.** muscle contraction

a. type of energy pathway used to produce ATP for muscle contractions

b. thin protein filament found in muscle tissue

c. thick protein filament in muscle found in tissue

d. time during which actin filaments and myosin filaments slide against one another

e. energy used to power muscle contractions

Name ______________________________ Class ______________ Date ____________

Skills Worksheet

Directed Reading

Section: Skin, Hair, and Nails

Complete each statement by writing the correct term or phrase in the space provided.

1. The outermost layer of the skin is the ________________________ .

2. The protein that makes skin tough and waterproof is ____________________ .

3. The outermost layer of skin cells is constantly being ____________________ .

4. A person's skin color is determined by the amount of

________________________ in the skin cells.

5. The ________________________ is the functional layer of skin.

6. Hair is produced by specialized structures called ________________________ .

Read each question, and write your answer in the space provided.

7. What are two ways the skin regulates body temperature?

____

____

8. Describe four functions of subcutaneous tissue.

____

____

Complete each statement by writing the correct term or phrase in the space provided.

9. Oil glands in the dermis release ________________________ , an oily secretion that lubricates the skin.

10. Acne is caused by excessive secretion from ________________________ glands.

Read each question, and write your answer in the space provided.

11. Distinguish between carcinomas and malignant melanomas.

____

____

12. What causes skin cancer?

____

Name ______________________ Class ______________ Date ____________

Skills Worksheet

Active Reading

Section: Body Organization

Read the passage below. Then answer the questions that follow.

Epithelial tissue: Epithelial tissue lines most body surfaces, and it protects other tissues from dehydration and physical damage. An epithelial layer is usually no more than a few cells thick. The cells are typically flat and thin and have only a small amount of cytoplasm. Epithelial tissue is constantly being replaced as cells die.

Nervous tissue: The nervous system is made of **nervous tissue.** Nervous tissue consists of nerve cells and their supporting cells. Nerve cells carry information throughout the body.

Connective tissue: Various types of **connective tissue** support, protect, and insulate the body. Connective tissue includes fat, cartilage, bone, tendons, and blood. Some connective tissue cells, such as those in bone, are densely packed. Others, such as those found in blood, are farther apart from each other.

Muscle tissue: Three kinds of **muscle tissue** enable the movement of body structures by muscle contractions. The three kinds of muscle tissues are skeletal muscle, smooth muscle, and cardiac muscle.

1. **Skeletal muscle** is considered voluntary muscle because you can consciously control its contractions. Skeletal muscles move bones in the trunk and limbs.
2. **Smooth muscle** is called involuntary muscle because you cannot consciously control its slow, long-lasting contractions. Some smooth muscles, such as those lining the walls of blood vessels, contract only when stimulated by signal molecules. Other smooth muscles contract spontaneously.
3. **Cardiac muscle** is found in the heart. The powerful, rhythmic contractions of cardiac muscle pump blood to all body tissues. Cardiac muscle consists of interconnected cells. Groups of neighboring cells contract all at once, stimulating adjacent groups of cells to contract.

SKILL: READING EFFECTIVELY

Read each question, and write your answer in the space provided.

1. Compare the concentration of connective tissue cells found in bone with the concentration of those found in blood.

____

____

2. Compare voluntary and involuntary muscle.

____

____

SKILL: RECOGNIZING SIMILARITIES AND DIFFERENCES

Identify the type of body tissue described. Write *epithelial tissue, nervous tissue, connective tissue, skeletal muscle, smooth muscle,* or *cardiac muscle* in the space provided.

________________________ **3.** its slow, long-lasting contractions cannot consciously be controlled

________________________ **4.** carries information throughout the body

________________________ **5.** moves bones in the trunk and limbs

________________________ **6.** lines most body surfaces

________________________ **7.** insulates the body

________________________ **8.** is found in the heart

________________________ **9.** protects other tissues from dehydration

________________________ **10.** holds structures together

________________________ **11.** is constantly being replaced as cells die

________________________ **12.** is made of nerve cells and their supporting cells

________________________ **13.** pumps blood to all body tissues

In the space provided, write the letter of the term or phrase that best completes the statement.

______ **14.** Fat, cartilage, bone, and tendons are types of

a. nervous tissue.
b. cardiac muscle.
c. epithelial tissue.
d. connective tissue.

Name ______________________________ Class ______________ Date ____________

Skills Worksheet

Active Reading

Section: Skeletal System

Read the passage below. Then answer the questions that follow.

Bones are made of a hard outer covering of compact bone surrounding a porous inner core of spongy bone. Compact bone is a dense connective tissue that provides a great deal of support. Spongy bone is a loosely structured network of separated connective tissue. Some cavities in spongy bone are filled with a soft tissue called **bone marrow.** Red bone marrow begins the production of all blood cells and platelets. The hollow interior of long bones is filled with yellow bone marrow. Yellow bone marrow consists mostly of fat, which stores energy. Bones are surrounded and protected by a tough exterior membrane called the **periosteum.** The periosteum contains many blood vessels that supply nutrients to bones.

SKILL: READING EFFECTIVELY

Read each question, and write your answer in the space provided.

1. Where does the production of blood cells and platelets begin?

____

____

2. What does yellow bone marrow consist of?

____

____

3. What does the periosteum supply to bones?

____

____

SKILL: INTERPRETING GRAPHICS

Label the following parts of the diagram: *bone marrow, compact bone, periosteum,* and *spongy bone.*

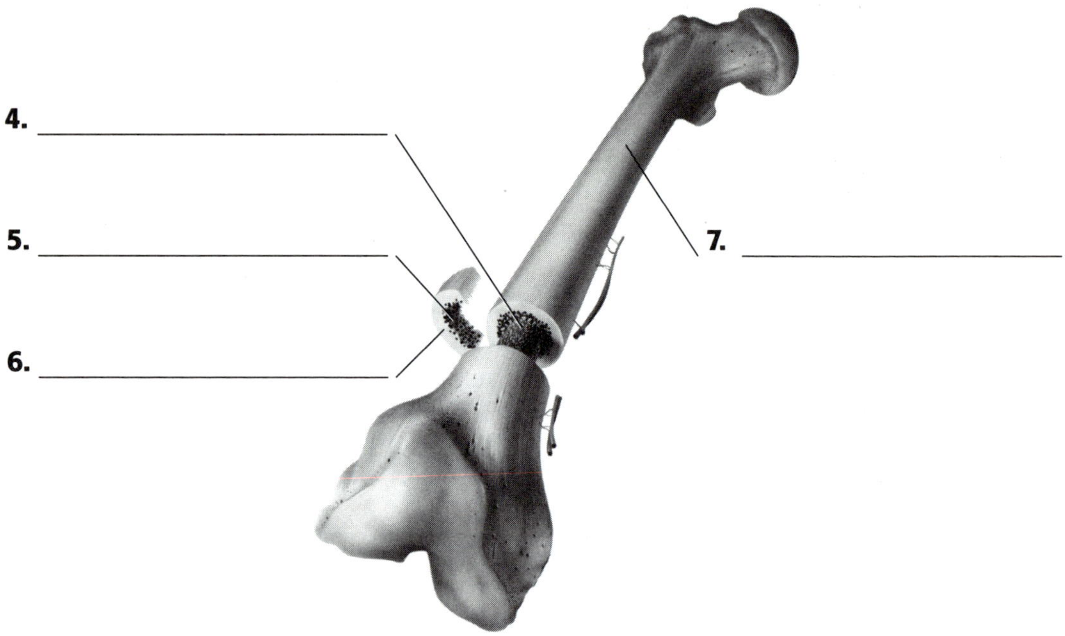

In the spaces provided, describe the differences between compact bone and spongy bone.

8. Compact bone: ____

9. Spongy bone: ____

In the space provided, write the letter of the term or phrase that best completes the statement.

______**10.** The interior of long bones is filled with yellow bone marrow, which consists mostly of

a. nervous tissue.
b. energy-storing fat.
c. red blood cells.
d. platelets.

Name ______________________________ Class ______________ Date ____________

Skills Worksheet

Active Reading

Section: Muscular System

Read the passage below. Then answer the questions that follow.

Muscles contain some connective tissue, which holds muscle cells together and provides elasticity. Muscle tissue also contains large amounts of protein filaments. These protein filaments, called **actin** and **myosin,** enable muscles to contract. Other characteristics of muscle tissue include the ability to stretch or expand and the ability to respond to stimuli, such as signal molecules released by nerve cells.

Skeletal muscle tissue consists of many parallel, elongated cells called muscle fibers. Each muscle fiber is made of small cylindrical structures called **myofibrils.** Myofibrils have alternating light and dark bands that produce a characteristic striated, or striped, appearance when viewed under a microscope. In the center of each light band is a structure called a Z line, which anchors actin filaments. The area between two Z lines is called a **sarcomere.** Thus, a myofibril is a grouping of sarcomeres linked end to end. Each sarcomere contains overlapping thin and thick protein filaments that move and interact with each other. The thin filaments are actin, and the thick filaments are myosin.

SKILL: READING EFFECTIVELY

Read each question, and write your answer in the space provided.

1. What is the function of the connective tissue found in muscle tissue, as described in the first sentence of the passage?

____

____

2. How are actin and myosin similar?

____

____

3. What effect do signal molecules released by nerve cells have on muscle tissue?

____

____

SKILL: INTERPRETING GRAPHICS

The figure illustrates the structure of a skeletal muscle. Label the following parts of the figure: *actin, myofibril, myosin, sarcomere,* and *Z line.*

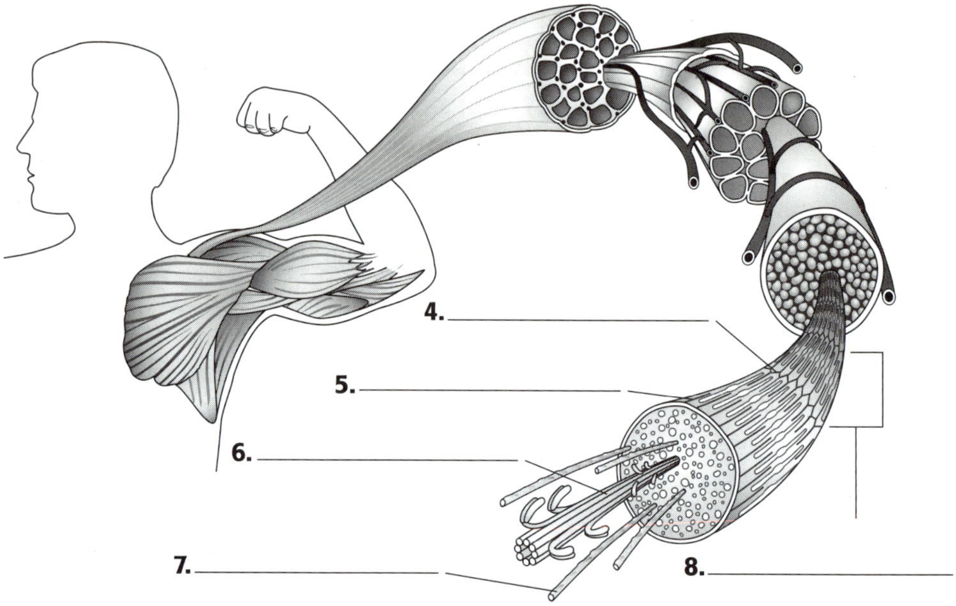

In the spaces provided, define the skeletal muscle parts listed in the figure above.

9. Actin: ________________________________

____

10. Myofibril: ________________________________

____

11. Myosin: ________________________________

____

12. Sarcomere: ________________________________

____

13. Z line: ________________________________

____

In the space provided, write the letter of the term or phrase that best completes the statement.

______**14.** Muscle tissue contains

a. protein filaments.
b. connective tissue.
c. white blood cells.
d. Both (a) and (b)

Name ______________________________ Class ______________ Date ____________

Skills Worksheet

Active Reading

Section: Skin, Hair, and Nails

Read the passage below. Then answer the questions that follow.

The most common skin problem for teenagers is acne, a chronic inflammatory condition that involves the skin's oil-producing glands. Oil glands in the dermis release **sebum,** an oily secretion that lubricates the skin. Sebum is released through ducts, or pores, into nearby hair follicles. These oil glands are especially active during adolescence. Acne is caused by excessive secretion of sebum, which blocks pores with oil, dirt, and bacteria. Makeup and other cosmetic products can contribute to clogging. As a result, the surrounding tissue becomes infected and inflamed, and the pores accumulate pus, producing pimples. Serious acne may need to be treated using antibiotics. Although acne cannot be prevented, it can usually be managed with proper skin care.

SKILL: READING EFFECTIVELY

Read each question, and write your answer in the space provided.

1. What word is defined in the first sentence of the passage? What does this word mean?

____

____

2. What Key Term is defined in the second sentence? What does this word mean?

____

____

3. What synonym for *ducts* is provided in the third sentence?

____

____

In the space provided, write the letter of the term or phrase that best completes the statement.

______ **4.** Sebum blocks pores with all of the following EXCEPT

a. pus.
b. dirt.
c. bacteria.
d. oil.

Name ______________________ Class ______________ Date ______________

Skills Worksheet

Vocabulary Review

In the space provided, write the letter of the description that best matches the term or phrase.

______ **1.** epithelial tissue

______ **2.** nervous tissue

______ **3.** muscle tissue

______ **4.** connective tissue

______ **5.** body cavities

a. carries information throughout the body

b. provides support, protection, and insulation

c. fluid-filled spaces that contain major body organs

d. enables the movement of body structures

e. lines most body surfaces

Complete each statement by writing the correct term or phrase in the space provided.

6. The ______________ ______________ includes bones of the skull, spine, ribs, and sternum.

7. The ______________ ______________ includes bones of the arms, legs, pelvis, and shoulder.

8. Bone ______________ is soft tissue inside bones that begins the manufacture of blood cells.

9. Bones are surrounded by a tough exterior membrane called the ______________ that contains blood vessels that supply nutrients to bones.

10. Hollow channels that contain blood vessels that enter bone through the periosteum are called ______________ ______________ .

11. Bone cells called ______________ maintain the mineral content of bone.

12. A disease that results in brittle bones and that affects more women than men is ______________ , meaning "brittle bone."

13. A junction between two or more bones is called a(n) ______________ .

14. Bones of a joint are held together by strong bands of connective tissue called ______________ .

Use the terms from the list below to fill in the blanks in the following passage.

actin	myofibrils	sarcomere
extensor	myosin	tendons
flexor		

Most skeletal muscles are attached to bones by strips of dense connective tissue called **(15)** ______________________ . One muscle in a pair of muscles pulls a bone in one direction, and the other muscle pulls the bone in the opposite direction. A(n) **(16)** ______________________ muscle causes a joint to bend, and a(n) **(17)** ______________________ muscle causes a joint to straighten.

Muscle tissue contains large amounts of protein filaments called **(18)** ______________________ and **(19)** ______________________ , which enable muscles to contract. Each muscle fiber is made of small cylindrical structures called **(20)** ______________________ , which have alternating light and dark bands when viewed under a microscope. In the center of each light band is a Z line, which anchors actin filaments. The area between the two Z lines is called a(n) **(21)** ______________________ , the functional unit of muscle contraction.

In the space provided, write the letter of the description that best matches the term or phrase.

______**22.** epidermis

______**23.** keratin

______**24.** melanin

______**25.** dermis

______**26.** subcutaneous tissue

______**27.** hair follicle

______**28.** sebum

a. protein that makes skin tough and waterproof

b. functional layer of skin that lies just beneath the epidermis

c. the outermost layer of skin

d. oily secretion that lubricates the skin

e. made mostly of fat

f. pigment that helps determine skin color

g. produces individual hairs

Name ______________________________ Class ______________ Date ____________

Skills Worksheet

Science Skills

INTERPRETING GRAPHICS

Use the figure below to answer questions 1–4.

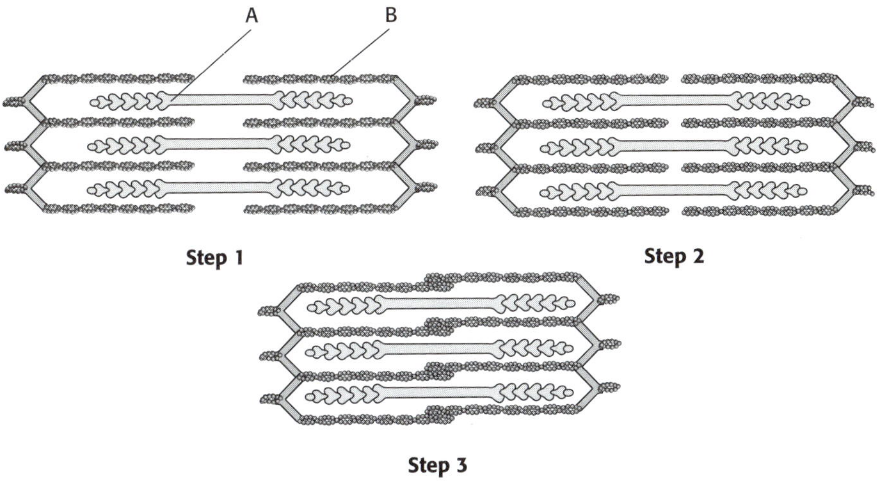

Read each question, and write your answer in the space provided.

1. The striped pattern of a sarcomere is formed by two different protein filaments, labeled *A* and *B*. Identify and briefly describe these two filaments.

____

____

____

2. How do these two protein filaments interact during muscle contraction?

____

____

3. Explain what is occurring in Step 2.

____

____

____

____

4. What substance is needed to go from Step 3 back to Step 1? Explain.

____

____

In the space provided, write the letter of each labeled bone in the figure below that matches the name of each bone.

______ **5.** fibula

______ **6.** ulna

______ **7.** pelvic girdle

______ **8.** scapula

______ **9.** sternum

______ **10.** vertebra

______ **11.** femur

______ **12.** carpals

______ **13.** metatarsals

______ **14.** patella

______ **15.** humerus

______ **16.** skull

______ **17.** metacarpals

______ **18.** tibia

______ **19.** radius

______ **20.** clavicle

______ **21.** tarsals

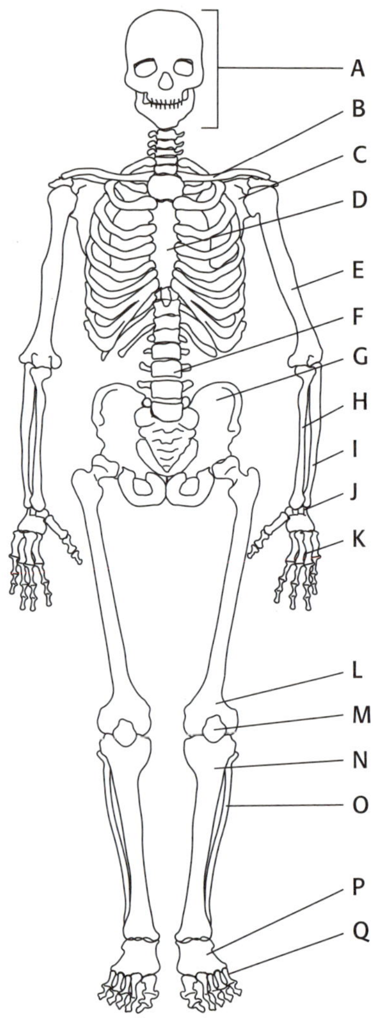

Read each question, and write your answer in the space provided.

22. What are the primary functions of the skeleton?

____

____

____

23. Distinguish between the axial skeleton and the appendicular skeleton.

____

____

____

Name ______________________ Class ______________ Date ____________

Skills Worksheet

Concept Mapping

Using the terms and phrases provided below, complete the concept map showing the organization of body structures.

appendicular skeleton	epithelial tissue	nervous tissue	skeletal muscle
axial skeleton	hair	organ systems	skin
cardiac muscle	muscular system	organs	
connective tissue	nails	pancreas	

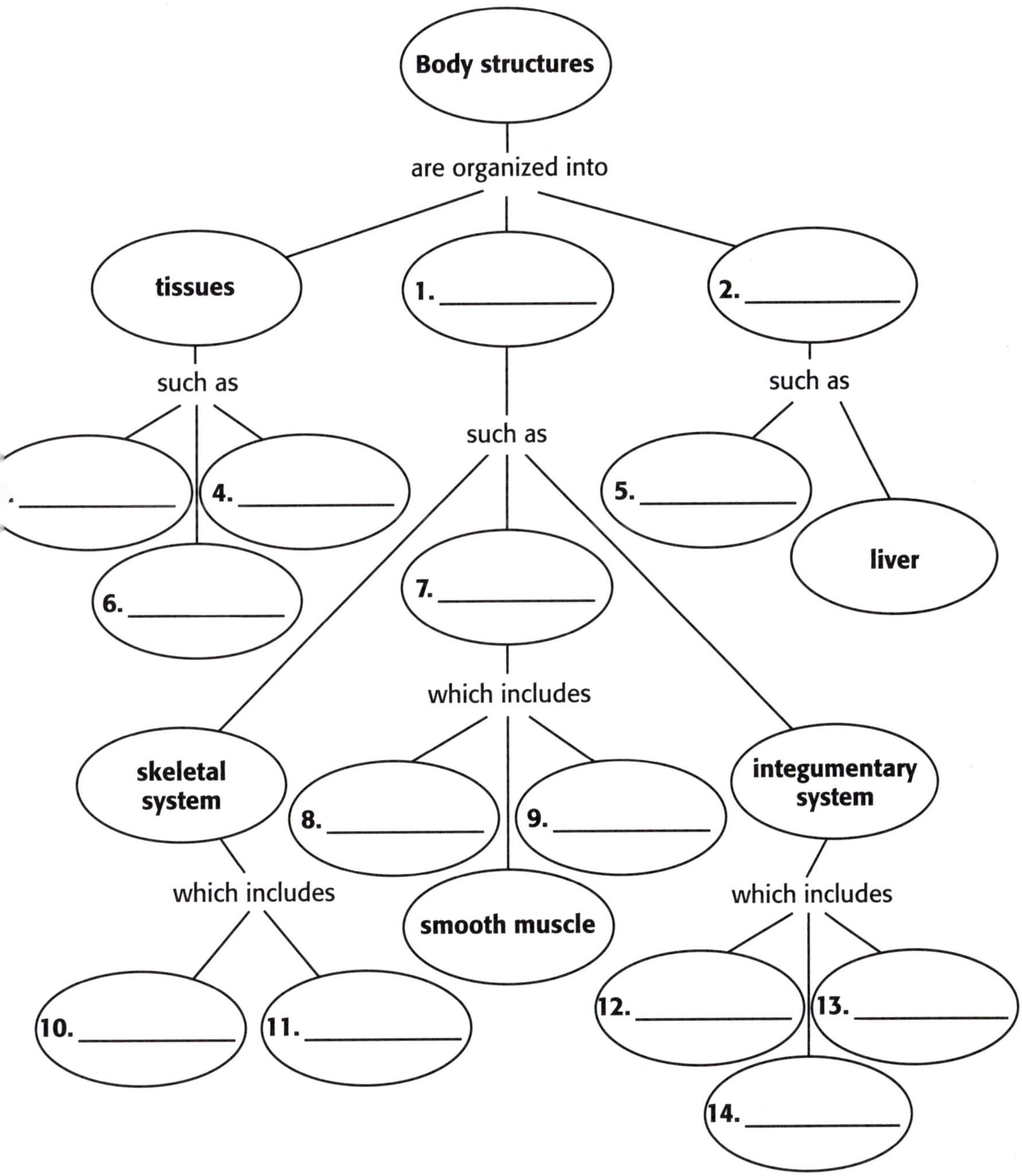

Name ______________________ Class ______________ Date ______________

Skills Worksheet

Critical Thinking

Look-Alikes

In the space provided, write the letter of the term or phrase that best describes how each numbered item looks.

______ **1.** concentric rings of compact bone

______ **2.** ribs and sternum

______ **3.** sweat glands

______ **4.** muscle fibers

______ **5.** spongy bone

a. growth rings on a tree trunk

b. bundle of uncooked spaghetti

c. cage

d. Swiss cheese

e. coiled snake

Work-Alikes

In the space provided, write the letter of the term or phrase that best describes how each numbered item functions.

______ **6.** cartilage pads in joints

______ **7.** ossified cartilage due to rheumatoid arthritis

______ **8.** epithelial tissue

______ **9.** ATP consumption exceeds ATP production during exercise

______ **10.** endothermy

a. mortar between bricks

b. running out of gas

c. thermostat on a furnace

d. protective padding for football players

e. shingles on a rooftop

Cause and Effect

In the space provided, write the letter of the term or phrase that best matches each cause or effect given below.

Cause	Effect
11. overextension of a ligament	______________
12. flexor muscle activity	______________
13. ______________	anaerobic respiration becomes the only source of ATP
14. aerobic exercise	______________

a. joint bends

b. increased muscle endurance

c. inadequate oxygen supply in rapidly contracting muscles

d. sports injury

Linkages

In the spaces provided, write the letters of the two terms or phrases that are linked together by the term or phrase in the middle. The choices can be placed in any order.

15. ______ blood vessels in Haversian canals ______

16. ______ increased bone density ______

17. ______ slightly movable ______

18. ______ smooth ______

19. ______ muscle ______

20. ______ evaporation ______

21. ______ clogged oil glands in skin ______

a. increased activity of adolescent oil glands

b. less likely to be affected by osteoporosis

c. acne

d. oxygen and nourishment

e. osteocytes

f. muscular insertion

g. regular exercise and mineral-rich diet

h. heat dissipation

i. muscle origin

j. sweat on skin surface

k. immovable

l. cardiac

m. freely movable

n. skeletal

Analogies

An analogy is a relationship between two pairs of terms or phrases written as a : b :: c : d. The symbol : is read as "is to," and the symbol :: is read as "as." In the space provided, write the letter of the pair of terms or phrases that best completes the analogy shown.

______**22.** Haversian canal : blood vessels ::

a. nerve cell : muscle tissue
b. muscle : bone tissue
c. tendon : muscle tissue
d. body : body cavities

______**23.** price tag : item of clothing ::

a. rib cage : pelvic girdle
b. appendicular skeleton : axial skeleton
c. cranium : sternum
d. pelvic girdle : ribs

______**24.** blood cells : bone marrow ::

a. bone cells : bone marrow
b. bone marrow : osteocytes
c. hair: hair follicle
d. bone cells : osteocytes

______**25.** muscle fiber : myofibrils ::

a. myofibril : actin and myosin
b. sarcomere : muscle fibers
c. actin : myosin
d. myosin : myofibrils

Name ______________________ Class ______________ Date ____________

Skills Worksheet

Test Prep Pretest

In the space provided, write the letter of the term or phrase that best completes each statement or best answers each question.

______ **1.** From simplest to most complex, the four levels of structural organization of the human body are as follows:
a. tissues, cells, organs, organ systems
b. cells, tissues, organs, organ systems
c. organ systems, tissues, cells, organs
d. cells, organs, tissues, organ systems

______ **2.** Types of connective tissue include all of the following EXCEPT
a. blood.
b. bone.
c. fat.
d. muscle.

______ **3.** Which of the following would likely occur if endothermy were disrupted?
a. Body temperature could not be maintained.
b. Strenuous physical activity would be difficult.
c. Enzymes would be inactivated.
d. All of the above

______ **4.** The appendicular skeleton includes bones of the
a. cranium.
b. spine.
c. pelvis.
d. ribs.

______ **5.** In early development, bone tissue is made mostly of
a. groups of osteocytes.
b. bone marrow.
c. periosteum.
d. cartilage.

In the space provided, write the letter of the description that best matches the term or phrase.

______ **6.** compact bone
______ **7.** spongy bone
______ **8.** red bone marrow
______ **9.** yellow bone marrow
______ **10.** periosteum
______ **11.** cartilage
______ **12.** Haversian canals
______ **13.** osteocytes

a. maintain mineral content of bone
b. template tissue for bone formation
c. site of blood cell production
d. channels containing blood vessels in concentric rings of compact bone
e. dense bone that provides a great deal of support
f. tough membrane surrounding bones
g. site of fat storage
h. loosely structured bone

Complete each statement by writing the correct term or phrase in the space provided.

14. The excretory system includes the kidneys, ______________________

______________________ , ureters, and the ______________________ .

15. Osteoporosis can be delayed or prevented by ______________________ and a diet containing ample ______________________ .

16. A muscle fiber contains many bundles of cylindrical structures called ______________________ .

17. When oxygen is plentiful, the ATP used to power muscle contractions is supplied by ______________________ processes. As oxygen becomes depleted, ATP is supplied by ______________________ processes.

18. A pigment found in the epidermis, ______________________ , absorbs UV radiation and helps determine skin color.

19. Hair consists mostly of dead cells filled with the protein called ______________________, the same protein that makes the skin tough and waterproof.

20. The dermis contains ______________________ ______________________ , which help regulate body temperature, either by radiating heat into the air or by helping to insulate the body.

21. The most common type of skin cancer originates in cells of the ______________________ that do not produce pigments.

22. Acne is caused by excessive secretion of ______________________ , an oily secretion that lubricates the skin, by oil glands.

Read each question, and write your answer in the space provided.

23. Describe the three main types of joints, and give an example of each.

24. Describe the interaction of myosin and actin during a muscle contraction.

25. Differentiate between the epidermis, the dermis, and subcutaneous tissue.

Name ______________________ Class ______________ Date ____________

Assessment

Quiz

Section: Body Organization

In the space provided, write the letter of the description that best matches the term or phrase.

______ **1.** stem cells

______ **2.** organ system

______ **3.** epithelial tissue

______ **4.** body cavities

______ **5.** endothermy

a. large fluid-filled spaces that house and protect the major internal organs

b. protects other tissues from dehydration and physical damage

c. early, undifferentiated cells that give rise to all types of cells of the developing body

d. maintaining a near-constant internal body temperature

e. group of organs that work together to carry out major processes

In the space provided, write the letter of the term or phrase that best completes each statement or best answers each question.

______ **6.** The nervous system consists of which of the following organs?
a. stomach, liver, pancreas
b. lungs, nose, trachea
c. kidneys, ureters, urinary bladder
d. brain, spinal cord, sense organs

______ **7.** Cell is to tissue as
a. cell is to organ system.
b. tissue is to organ.
c. organ system is to tissue.
d. organ system is to organ.

______ **8.** The function of cardiac muscle tissue is to
a. move bones in the trunk and limbs.
b. support, protect, and insulate the body.
c. carry information throughout the body.
d. pump blood to all muscle tissues.

______ **9.** Which of the following organs is found in the cranial cavity?
a. stomach
b. spinal cord
c. brain
d. heart

______**10.** A function of the respiratory system is to
a. control gas exchange between the blood and lungs.
b. extract and absorb nutrients from food.
c. defend against pathogens and disease.
d. help regulate body temperature.

Name ______________________ Class ______________ Date ____________

Assessment

Quiz

Section: Skeletal System

In the space provided, write the letter of the description that best matches the term or phrase.

______ **1.** appendicular skeleton

______ **2.** Haversian canal

______ **3.** osteocyte

______ **4.** axial skeleton

______ **5.** joint

a. hollow channel that contains blood vessels, found in compact bone

b. place where two bones meet

c. includes bones of the arms, legs, pelvis, and shoulder

d. cell imbedded in bone tissue, which maintains the mineral content of bone

e. includes bones of the skull, spine, ribs, and sternum

In the space provided, write the letter of the term or phrase that best completes each statement or best answers each question.

______ **6.** A joint that permits limited movement of the bones it joins is called a(n)

a. freely movable joint.
b. immovable joint.
c. slightly movable joint.
d. None of the above

______ **7.** The disorder that causes the degeneration of the cartilage that covers the surfaces of bones is called

a. osteoporosis.
b. rheumatoid arthritis.
c. osteoarthritis.
d. porous bones.

______ **8.** What are the functions of the skeletal system?

a. to support the body and protect internal organs
b. to transport nutrients and gases
c. to regulate body temperature and metabolism
d. to produce gametes and offspring

______ **9.** Red bone marrow produces

a. fat.
b. bone cells.
c. blood vessels.
d. blood cells and platelets.

______ **10.** Which of the following helps stabilize and prevent joints from moving too far in any one direction?

a. tendons
b. ligaments
c. cartilage
d. muscle

Name ______________________ Class ______________ Date ____________

Assessment

Quiz

Section: Muscular System

In the space provided, write the letter of the description that best matches the term or phrase.

______ **1.** actin

______ **2.** myosin

______ **3.** myofibril

______ **4.** sarcomere

______ **5.** ATP

a. the area between two Z lines

b. energy used to power muscle contractions

c. thin protein filament found in muscle tissue

d. small, cylindrical structures within a muscle fiber

e. thick protein filament found in muscle tissue

In the space provided, write the letter of the term or phrase that best completes each statement or best answers each question.

______ **6.** The opposing pairs of muscles involved in the movement of limbs are called

a. tendons and ligaments.
b. flexors and extensors.
c. myofibrils and sarcomeres.
d. actin and myosin.

______ **7.** A muscle contraction begins when

a. a sarcomere is fully contracted.
b. a myosin head detaches from an actin filament.
c. a muscle fiber is stimulated by a nerve cell.
d. ATP binds to actin.

______ **8.** Muscle fatigue and soreness may result when

a. ATP consumption equals ATP production.
b. ATP consumption is less than ATP production.
c. ATP consumption exceeds ATP production.
d. None of the above

______ **9.** Which of the following lists the components of muscle tissue in the correct order from smallest to largest?

a. actin and myosin filaments, myofibril, sarcomere
b. sarcomere, muscle fiber, myofibril
c. myofibril, muscle fiber, actin and myosin filaments
d. actin and myosin filaments, sarcomere, myofibril

______ **10.** The bone that remains stationary during a muscle contraction is called the

a. origin.
b. flexor.
c. insertion.
d. extensor.

Name ______________________ Class ______________ Date ____________

Assessment

Quiz

Section: Skin, Hair, and Nails

In the space provided, write the letter of the description that best matches the term or phrase.

______ **1.** subcutaneous tissue

______ **2.** keratin

______ **3.** melanin

______ **4.** sebum

______ **5.** epidermis

a. pigment that absorbs UV radiation

b. layer of connective tissue made mostly of fat

c. protein that makes skin tough and waterproof

d. outermost layer of skin

e. an oily secretion that lubricates the skin

In the space provided, write the letter of the term or phrase that best completes each statement or best answers each question.

______ **6.** Which of the following structures are NOT found in the dermis?
a. nerve cells
b. hair follicles
c. blood vessels
d. cells that produce melanin

______ **7.** Skin cancer is to exposure to UV radiation as
a. tendon is to tendonitis.
b. acne is to excessive secretion of sebum.
c. lack of exercise is to osteoporosis.
d. rheumatoid arthritis is to freely movable joints.

______ **8.** Which of the following structures or substance is NOT found in epidermis?
a. keratin
b. hair
c. sweat gland
d. pore

______ **9.** Which of the following structures helps remove excess heat from the body?
a. hair
b. nerve cell
c. subcutaneous tissue
d. sweat gland

______ **10.** The functions of the skin include
a. protecting the body against injury, infection, and fluid loss.
b. producing red blood cells.
c. controlling sensory and motor systems.
d. transporting nutrients.

Name ______________________ Class ______________ Date ____________

Assessment

Chapter Test

Introduction to Body Structure

In the space provided, write the letter of the term or phrase that best completes each statement or best answers each question.

______ **1.** The main components of the epidermis are
a. epithelial tissue and nervous tissue.
b. connective tissue and muscle tissue.
c. connective tissue and epithelial tissue.
d. nervous tissue and muscle tissue.

______ **2.** Which of the following structures causes a joint to straighten?
a. tendon
b. ligament
c. extensor
d. flexor

______ **3.** A group of similar cells that work together to perform a common function is
a. an organ.
b. an organ system.
c. a cell.
d. a tissue.

______ **4.** Which of the following sets of bones are part of the axial skeleton?
a. skull, legs, hips
b. vertebrae, skull, arms
c. skull, vertebrae, sternum
d. ribs, legs, arms

______ **5.** Hair and nails are derived from cells of the
a. dermis.
b. subcutaneous tissue.
c. oil glands.
d. epidermis.

______ **6.** When a sarcomere is fully contracted,
a. myosin and actin completely overlap each other.
b. the sarcomere is at its longest length.
c. myosin and actin are not connected at all.
d. ATP is not being used.

______ **7.** Which of the following is the correct order of structures that compose a bone from the outermost structure to the innermost structure?
a. periosteum, bone marrow, compact bone, spongy bone
b. periosteum, compact bone, spongy bone, bone marrow
c. compact bone, spongy bone, bone marrow, periosteum
d. spongy bone, periosteum, compact bone, bone marrow

______ **8.** The structures in the dermis that help regulate body temperature are
a. hair follicles and blood vessels.
b. blood vessels and sweat glands.
c. oil glands and sweat glands.
d. nerve cells and blood vessels.

______ **9.** The functions of the skin include all of the following EXCEPT
a. protecting the body from injury.
b. preventing the body from drying out.
c. protecting the body from infection.
d. absorbing nutrients from food.

______ **10.** Energy for muscle contraction can be supplied by
a. aerobic processes.
b. anaerobic processes.
c. glycolysis.
d. All of the above

______ **11.** Eating a mineral-rich diet and exercising regularly can help prevent which of the following disorders?
a. rheumatoid arthritis
b. malignant melanoma
c. osteoporosis
d. osteoarthritis

______ **12.** Which of the following tissue types enables the movement of body structures?
a. nervous tissue
b. epithelial tissue
c. muscle tissue
d. connective tissue

______ **13.** Which of the following is NOT part of the immune system?
a. heart
b. lymph nodes
c. skin
d. white blood cells

______ **14.** Disorders of the skin include all of the following EXCEPT
a. acne.
b. osteoporosis.
c. malignant melanomas.
d. carcinomas.

______ **15.** Endothermy is important because it enables organisms to
a. remain active at external temperatures that would slow the activity of ectoderms.
b. sustain strenuous activity for a long period of time.
c. maintain a body temperature in which enzymes will not be inactivated.
d. All of the above

Questions 16–20 refer to the figure below, which shows three different joints. In the space provided, write the letter of each joint that best matches the term or phrase. Some choices may be used more than once.

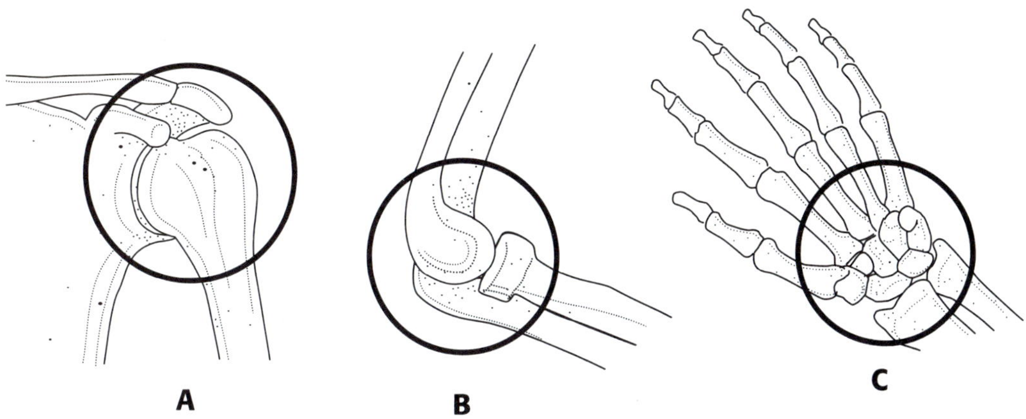

______ **16.** ball and socket joint

______ **17.** gliding joint

______ **18.** hinge joint

______ **19.** joint also found in the ankles

______ **20.** joint also found in the hip

Name ________________ Class ________________ Date ________________

Assessment

Chapter Test

Introduction to Body Structure

In the space provided, write the letter of the term or phrase that best completes each statement or best answers each question.

______ **1.** The condition in which bone density is lost and bones become brittle is called
- **a.** ossification.
- **b.** osteoporosis.
- **c.** rheumatoid arthritis.
- **d.** tendonitis.

______ **2.** Which of the following is NOT a hinge joint?
- **a.** elbow
- **b.** wrist
- **c.** finger knuckle
- **d.** toe knuckle

______ **3.** Each organ belongs to at least one
- **a.** tissue.
- **b.** organ system.
- **c.** muscle group.
- **d.** body cavity.

Questions 4 and 5 refer to the figure below, which shows the structure of the skin.

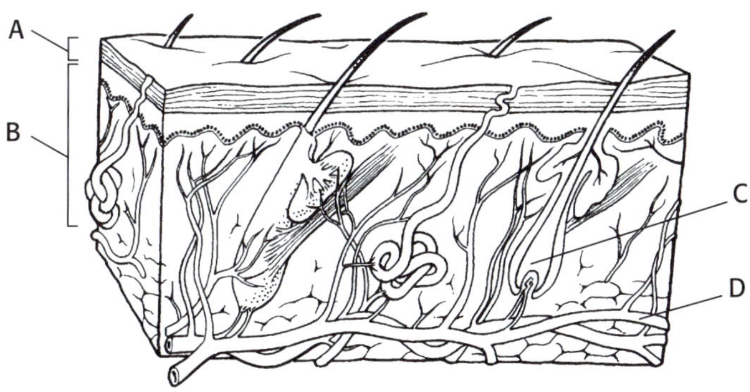

______ **4.** The epidermis is the structure labeled
- **a.** *A.*
- **b.** *B.*
- **c.** *C.*
- **d.** *D.*

______ **5.** The functional layer of the skin is labeled
- **a.** *A.*
- **b.** *B.*
- **c.** *C.*
- **d.** *D.*

______ **6.** Smooth muscle is also called
a. rhythmic muscle.
b. voluntary muscle.
c. interconnected muscle.
d. involuntary muscle.

______ **7.** The heart is part of which organ system?
a. nervous system
b. reproductive system
c. skeletal system
d. circulatory system

Complete each statement by writing the correct term or phrase in the space provided.

8. The body maintains a constant temperature because of ______________, which enables homeostasis.

9. The bones of the skull, spine, and rib cage make up the ______________ ______________ ______________.

10. Muscles that cause a joint to bend are called ______________.

11. The ATP used to power muscle contractions is supplied by aerobic processes when ______________ is plentiful. As ______________ becomes depleted, ATP is supplied by anaerobic processes.

12. Hair is produced by ______________ ______________.

13. Cells that are not yet specialized and that can divide indefinitely are called ______________ ______________ ______________.

In the space provided, write the letter of the description that best matches the term or phrase.

______ **14.** osteoporosis
______ **15.** carcinoma
______ **16.** osteoarthritis
______ **17.** tendonitis
______ **18.** melanoma
______ **19.** rheumatoid arthritis
______ **20.** acne

a. skin disorder caused by excess production of sebum
b. type of skin cancer that originates in skin cells that do not produce pigments
c. type of skin cancer that originates in pigment-producing skin cells
d. inflammation of the tendons caused by excessive stress
e. disorder caused by loss of bone density
f. inflammation of freely movable joints
g. disorder that causes the degeneration of cartilage that covers the surfaces of bones

Read each question, and write your answer in the space provided.

21. Briefly describe the interaction of muscle filaments during muscle contraction.

____

____

____

____

22. What is the outermost layer of skin, and what is its function?

____

____

____

____

23. Describe how bone cells are nourished.

____

____

____

____

24. Describe how the dermis helps maintain homeostasis.

____

____

____

____

25. Briefly describe the causes of skin cancer. What can be done to prevent the development of skin cancer?

____

____

____

____

Name ______________________________ Class ______________ Date ____________

Exploration Lab

DATASHEET FOR IN-TEXT LAB

Analyzing the Work of Muscles

SKILLS

- Using scientific methods
- Data collection
- Data interpretation

OBJECTIVE

- **Relate** muscles to the work they do.
- **Observe** the effects of fatigue

MATERIALS

- watch with second hand
- graph paper
- spring hand grips

Before You Begin

Muscles are attached to bones. As muscles contract, they move the bones to which they are attached. This is a basic type of work accomplished by the human body. As muscles are used, lactic acid builds up, resulting in **fatigue.** In this lab you will investigate how fatigue affects the amount of work that muscles can do.

1. Write a definition for the boldface term in the preceding paragraph.

____

2. Use the data table below.

Data Table For Muscle Contractions

Number of Muscle Contractions in 10-Second Intervals

Time	1st 10 sec	2nd 10 sec	3rd 10 sec	4th 10 sec	5th 10 sec	6th 10 sec	7th 10 sec	8th 10 sec	9th 10 sec	10th 10 sec	11th 10 sec	12th 10 sec	13th 10 sec	14th 10 sec
Trial 1														
Trial 2														
Trial 3														
Trial 4														

PROCEDURE

1. Perform this investigation with a partner. Designate one laboratory partner to observe and record while the other performs the experiment.
2. Hold the spring hand grips in your left hand if you are right-handed, or in your right hand if you are left-handed. Squeeze the grips rapidly and as hard as possible at a steady pace, until complete fatigue is experienced in the muscles of your hand and forearm.
3. The recorder should count and record the number of squeezes for every 10 seconds.
4. Allow the experimenter to rest for 1 minute and repeat the procedure for two more trials.
5. Record the data in your table. Some spaces may be left blank.
6. Switch roles with your partner and repeat the procedure.

Analyze and Conclude

1. **Summarizing Results** Use graph paper to plot the results of the three trials on a graph. The x-axis should be used for time in seconds and the y-axis for the number of muscle contractions.
2. **Analyzing Data** Account for the differences in the amount of work done by the muscles during the three trials.

   ____

   ____

3. **Drawing Conclusions** What is the relationship between the work muscles can do and fatigue?

   ____

   ____

   ____

4. **Predicting Patterns** How does the work done in the muscles of your hands and arms relate to the work done by the muscle of your heart?

   ____

   ____

5. **Further Inquiry** Compare the charts and the graphs of the athletes and nonathletes.

   ____

   ____

Name ______________________ Class ______________ Date ____________

Quick Lab **OBSERVATION**

Comparing Skeletal Joints

The bones of your skeleton come together in joints. In this activity, you will explore the types of skeletal joints found in your body by observing an example of each type of joint and surveying the other joints in your body.

OBJECTIVES

Identify and **compare** skeletal joints.

MATERIALS

- human skull or other animal skull
- paper
- pen

Procedure

1. Use a separate sheet of paper to make a table for recording your observations of the skeletal joints shown in **Figure 1.** Leave space in your table to identify where each type of joint is found in the human body.

FIGURE 1 SKELETAL JOINTS

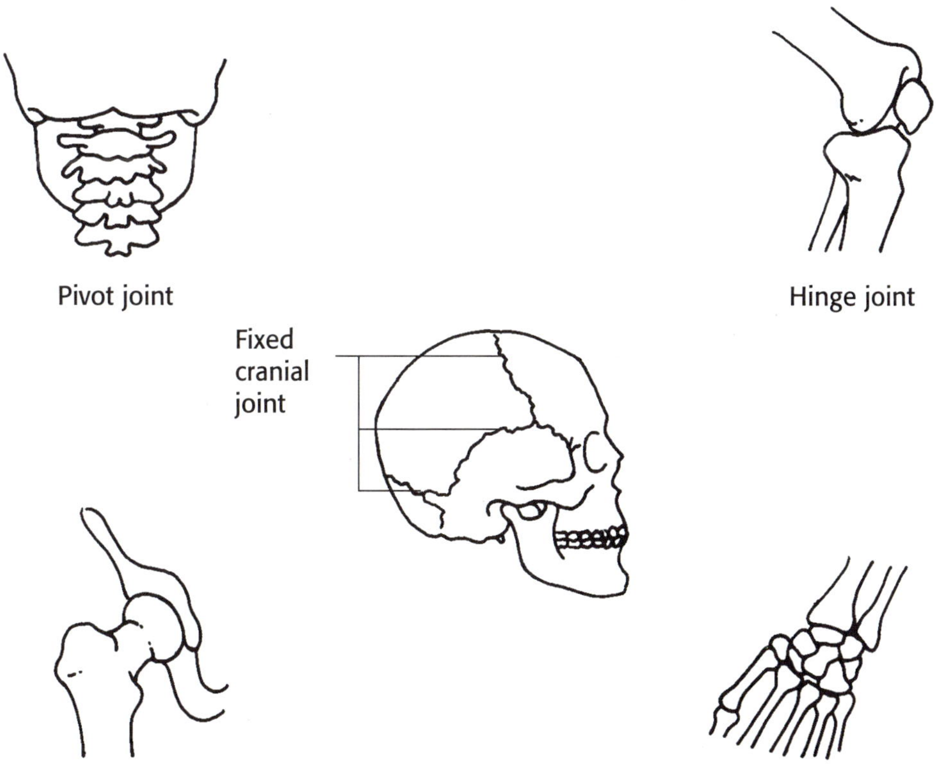

2. **CAUTION: Do not move in ways that can cause injury or pain.** Straighten your index finger as if to point. Slowly bend the finger until it touches your palm. Moving only your finger, try to move the individual parts of the finger in other directions. Record your description of the movements in your table by the type of joint present in the finger.
3. Move your arm in as many ways as possible. By the types of joints present in a shoulder and an elbow, record your description of the movements first from the shoulder, then from the elbow.
4. Place your hands on the sides of your neck to hold the neck in place. Gently move only your head in all possible directions. Try not to let your neck bend. Record your observations of the movements by the type of joint in the neck.
5. Use your left hand to grip your right arm just above the wrist. Without moving your forearm, move your hand in all possible directions. Record your observations of the movements after identifying the type of joint present in the wrist.
6. Examine the joints in the top of a skull. Gently press on each side of the joints to see if movement is possible without damaging the skull. Record your observations by the type of joint in the skull.
7. Starting with your feet, examine the movement of each of the other joints in your skeleton. Record the other locations in the body where you discover each type of joint.

Analysis and Conclusions

1. **Recognizing Patterns** Rank the five types of joints according to their freedom of movement. Start with the joint that allows the least freedom of movement.

____

____

2. **Identifying Relationships** Which types of joints are involved in walking?

____

____

3. **Applying Conclusions** For each type of skeletal joint, name a common, nonliving object that has a similar type of joint in its construction.

____

____

____

Name ______________________ Class ______________ Date ____________

Inquiry Lab

DESIGN YOUR OWN

Distribution of Touch Receptors

In this lab, you will design and conduct an experiment to compare the distribution of touch receptors in the skin among different parts of the body.

OBJECTIVES

Develop a hypothesis to compare the sensitivities of different areas of the body to touch stimuli.

Design and **conduct** an experiment to test your hypothesis.

Evaluate your results and recognize the need to reduce bias in experimentation.

POSSIBLE MATERIALS

- blindfold
- corrugated cardboard, 3 × 5 cm (7)
- metric ruler
- paper clips (13)
- tape

Finding Out More Information

Skin, the largest organ of the human body, is sensitive to touch, pain, heat, and cold. Tactile sensation, or touch, relies on different types of receptors. One type of receptor is located deep in the dermis, the thick, inner layer of the skin. This receptor responds to strong pressure. Another type is located just below the epidermis, the outermost layer of the skin. This type of receptor responds to light touch. Touch receptors are located throughout your skin over your entire body. However, some areas of your skin have more touch receptors per square centimeter than do other areas.

If the touch receptors in the skin are relatively sparse, two stimuli applied to the skin will stimulate only one touch receptor and, thus, be perceived as one stimulus. If the receptors are spaced closely, two stimuli applied to the skin will stimulate two receptors and, thus, be perceived as two stimuli.

1. Which areas of the skin are likely to be more sensitive than others, that is, have more touch receptors?

Procedure

FORMING A HYPOTHESIS

Based on what you have learned, form a hypothesis about which areas of the skin are more sensitive (have more touch receptors) than others.

1. How can you determine the sensitivity of a particular area of the skin?

____

____

____

____

2. How can you compare the relative sensitivities of different areas of the skin?

____

____

____

____

____

3. Write your hypothesis. A possible hypothesis might be "The skin on the calf is [more/less] sensitive than the skin on the palm, and the skin on the palm is [more/less] sensitive than the skin on the forearm.

____

____

COMING UP WITH A PLAN

Plan and conduct an experiment to compare how sensitive the skin is on various parts of the body.

4. Write out a procedure for your experiment on a separate sheet of paper. As you plan the procedure, make the following decisions.

- Decide which areas of the body you will test. Areas to consider include the fingers, calf, palm, forearm, upper arm, and neck.
- Decide how to construct a device (or devices) for stimulating the skin, using the materials provided or other materials that you choose.
- Decide on the number of trials you will run for each area of the body.

- Be sure to include a control that prevents the test subject from anticipating two stimuli and, therefore, guessing that two stimuli are present even when both are not felt. This type of response is referred to as bias because the subject's response may be based on the subject's expectation, rather than on the subject's observation. The possibility of bias exists when a person's subjective evaluation is required in an experiment. Bias can be difficult, but not impossible, to control.

5. Decide what safety procedures are necessary. Add them to your written procedure.

6. Using graph paper or a computer, construct tables to organize your data. Be sure that your data tables contain the appropriate information for the procedure you are following.

7. Have your teacher approve your plan.

PERFORMING THE EXPERIMENT

8. Implement your plan, using the equipment and safety procedures that you selected.

9. Record your data in your tables. If necessary, revise your tables to include variables that you did not think of while planning your experiment.

10. At the end of the experiment, pool the class data and determine the relative sensitivity of different areas of the body.

11. When you have finished, clean and store your equipment. Recycle or dispose of all materials as instructed by your teacher.

Analysis

SAMPLE TABLE

Distance between stimuli	Number of stimuli perceived					
	Calf		Palm		Forearm	
	Subject 1	Subject 2	Subject 1	Subject 2	Subject 1	Subject 2
1 stimulus						
2 mm						
5 mm	2	2				
10 mm			2	2		
20 mm						
30 mm					2	
40 mm						2

1. **Summarizing Data** What was the minimum distance between stimuli at which the test subject could consistently sense them as two points on the body parts you tested?

2. **Identifying/Recognizing Patterns** Relate your results to the number of skin receptors.

3. **Analyzing Data** Were there any differences between the data obtained for you and your partner? What could account for this?

Conclusions

1. **Drawing Conclusions** Based on your data, rank the areas of the body that you tested from most to least sensitive.

2. **Evaluating Methods** What was your control to minimize bias, that is, to keep the subject from guessing the number of stimuli being tested?

3. **Evaluating Methods** Besides the control in question 1, what other type of controls did you use, or could have used to minimize bias?

4. **Applying Conclusions** Describe a situation in which expectations could produce data that are in error.

____

____

5. **Applying Conclusions** What kinds of results would you expect if you were to test other body parts? Examples include the finger, lip, nose, foot, forehead, belly, upper arm, neck, shoulder and thigh. Give a reason for your answer.

____

____

____

____

____

____

____

____

____

____

Name ________________________ Class ______________ Date ______________

Exploration Lab

DATASHEET FOR IN-TEXT LAB

Analyzing the Work of Muscles

SKILLS

- Using scientific methods
- Data collection
- Data interpretation

OBJECTIVE

- **Relate** muscles to the work they do.
- **Observe** the effects of fatigue

MATERIALS

- watch with second hand
- graph paper
- spring hand grips

Before You Begin

Muscles are attached to bones. As muscles contract, they move the bones to which they are attached. This is a basic type of work accomplished by the human body. As muscles are used, lactic acid builds up, resulting in **fatigue.** In this lab you will investigate how fatigue affects the amount of work that muscles can do.

1. Write a definition for the bold face term in the preceding paragraph.

***Fatigue* means "to become tired."**

2. Use the data table below.

Data Table For Muscle Contractions														
Number of Muscle Contractions in 10-Second Intervals														
Time	1st 10 sec	2nd 10 sec	3rd 10 sec	4th 10 sec	5th 10 sec	6th 10 sec	7th 10 sec	8th 10 sec	9th 10 sec	10th 10 sec	11th 10 sec	12th 10 sec	13th 10 sec	14th 10 sec
Trial 1														
Trial 2														
Trial 3														
Trial 4														

PROCEDURE

1. Perform this investigation with a partner. Designate one laboratory partner to observe and record while the other performs the experiment.
2. Hold the spring hand grips in your left hand if you are right-handed, or in your right hand if you are left-handed. Squeeze the grips rapidly and as hard as possible at a steady pace, until complete fatigue is experienced in the muscles of your hand and forearm.
3. The recorder should count and record the number of squeezes for every 10 seconds.
4. Allow the experimenter to rest for one minute and repeat the procedure for two more trials.
5. Record the data in your table. Some spaces may be left blank.
6. Switch roles with your partner and repeat the procedure.

Analyze and Conclude

1. **Summarizing Results** Use graph paper to plot the results of the three trials on a graph. The x-axis should be used for time in seconds and the y-axis for the number of muscle contractions. **Number of muscle contractions probably decreases over time.**
2. **Analyzing Data** Account for the differences in the amount of work done by the muscles during the three trials.

   When muscles are fatigued, they can do less work than when they are not fatigued.
3. **Drawing Conclusions** What is the relationship between the work muscles can do and fatigue?

   The muscles have more energy, in the form of ATP, when they are first used, but the supply is quickly used and lactic acid is formed as a waste product. Time is needed for ATP molecules to re-form and lactic acid to dissipate.
4. **Predicting Patterns** How does the work done in the muscles of your hands and arms relate to the work done by the muscle of your heart?

   Both types of work involve muscles contracting. However, the heart muscle is able to contract regularly without fatigue because it rests between beats.
5. **Further Inquiry** Compare the charts and the graphs of the athletes and nonathletes.

   Answers may vary, but athletes may have muscles that show fatigue less quickly than nonatheletes.

Quick Lab

OBSERVATION

Comparing Skeletal Joints

Teacher Notes

TIME REQUIRED 20 minutes

SKILLS ACQUIRED

Collecting data
Experimenting
Identifying patterns
Recognizing patterns
Inferring
Interpreting
Measuring
Organizing and analyzing data

RATINGS Easy ← 1 2 3 4 → Hard

Teacher Prep–2
Student Setup-1
Concept Level-2
Cleanup-1

THE SCIENTIFIC METHOD

Make Observations The Procedure asks students to make and record observations.

Analyze the Results Analysis and Conclusions questions 1 and 2 require students to analyze their results.

Draw Conclusions Analysis and Conclusions question 3 requires students to draw conclusions from their data.

MATERIALS

Skulls for this lab activity can be purchased from WARD'S. See the *Master Materials List* for ordering instructions.

Have real or artificial skulls available to illustrate immovable or fixed joints. The skull of any animal can be substituted for a human skull. A detailed illustration will suffice if necessary.

If animal skulls are obtained from a butcher shop, be sure they have been boiled and all soft tissue removed.

DISPOSAL

Keep skulls for later use with other classes.

TECHNIQUES TO DEMONSTRATE

You might want to demonstrate Procedure steps 2–7 to emphasize that they should be done safely, without using unnecessary force that might harm joints or muscles.

TIPS AND TRICKS

Preparation

Advise students that this lab should be done individually, not with a lab partner.

Find out before beginning the lab whether any students have conditions or recent injuries that might restrict their movements. Allow these students to observe and record the movements of another student.

Procedure

Tell students to use common sense and care while making the movements described in the lab. Only normal movements are required. Review the procedure for examining the movement of the pivot joint. Holding the neck is necessary to illustrate the limited side-to-side movement of this joint.

Procedure Answers

2. Hinge joints allow the index finger to move in a forward and backward direction.
3. A ball-and-socket joint allows the wide movement between the arm and shoulder, whereas the elbow is a hinge joint with limited movement.
4. Rotating movement by a pivot joint allows the movement between the head and the neck.
5. Gliding joints allow movement of the wrist.
6. Fixed cranial joints allow no movement.
7. Some examples of different joints include the following:
   ball-and-socket: shoulders, hips
   pivot: top of spine (turning of head)
   hinge: elbows, knuckles of fingers and toes
   gliding: wrists, ankles

MISCONCEPTION ALERT

Many students associate joints with movement. Although this assumption is usually valid, emphasize that the cranial joints are examples of where bones are joined together but no movement occurs.

Name ______________________ Class ____________ Date ____________

Quick Lab **OBSERVATION**

Comparing Skeletal Joints

The bones of your skeleton come together in joints. In this activity, you will explore the types of skeletal joints found in your body by observing an example of each type of joint and surveying the other joints in your body.

OBJECTIVES

Identify and **compare** skeletal joints.

MATERIALS

- human skull or other animal skull
- paper
- pen

Procedure

1. Use a separate sheet of paper to make a table for recording your observations of the skeletal joints shown in **Figure 1.** Leave space in your table to identify where each type of joint is found in the human body.

FIGURE 1 SKELETAL JOINTS

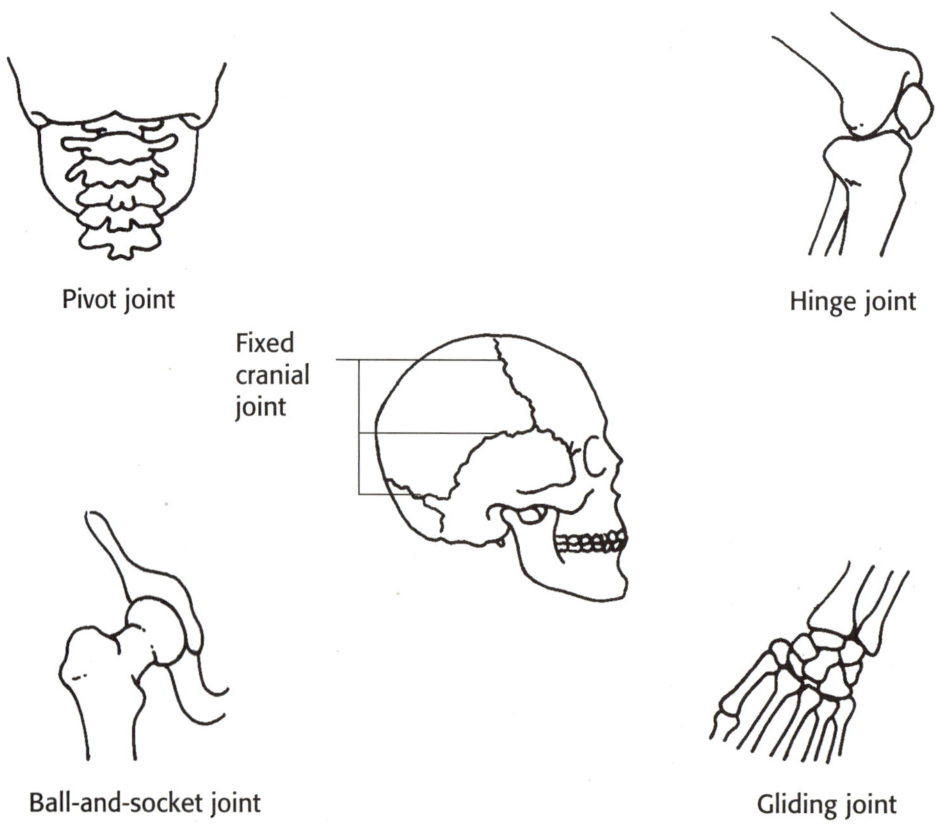

2. **CAUTION: Do not move in ways that can cause injury or pain.** Straighten your index finger as if to point. Slowly bend the finger until it touches your palm. Moving only your finger, try to move the individual parts of the finger in other directions. Record your description of the movements in your table by the type of joint present in the finger.
3. Move your arm in as many ways as possible. By the types of joints present in a shoulder and an elbow, record your description of the movements first from the shoulder, then from the elbow.
4. Place your hands on the sides of your neck to hold the neck in place. Gently move only your head in all possible directions. Try not to let your neck bend. Record your observations of the movements by the type of joint in the neck.
5. Use your left hand to grip your right arm just above the wrist. Without moving your forearm, move your hand in all possible directions. Record your observations of the movements after identifying the type of joint present in the wrist.
6. Examine the joints in the top of a skull. Gently press on each side of the joints to see if movement is possible without damaging the skull. Record your observations by the type of joint in the skull.
7. Starting with your feet, examine the movement of each of the other joints in your skeleton. Record the other locations in the body where you discover each type of joint.

Analysis and Conclusions

1. **Recognizing Patterns** Rank the five types of joints according to their freedom of movement. Start with the joint that allows the least freedom of movement.

   The joints are the fixed cranial joint, pivot joint, glide joint, hinge joint, and ball-and-socket joint.

2. **Identifying Relationships** Which types of joints are involved in walking?

   The joints involved in walking are the ball-and-socket joint, hinge joint, and glide joints.

3. **Applying Conclusions** For each type of skeletal joint, name a common, nonliving object that has a similar type of joint in its construction.

   Answers might include the expansion joint in bridges, a beacon, small disk or ball attached to the underside of furniture legs to allow easy sliding, door hinges, ball-and-socket wrenches, and lamps.

Name ______________________ Class ______________ Date ____________

Inquiry Lab

DESIGN YOUR OWN

Distribution of Touch Receptors

Teacher Notes

TIME REQUIRED One 45-minute period

SKILLS ACQUIRED

Collecting data
Designing experiments
Identifying and recognizing patterns
Interpreting
Measuring
Organizing and analyzing data

RATINGS

Easy ← 1 2 3 4 → Hard

Teacher Prep–1
Student Setup–2
Concept Level–3
Cleanup–1

THE SCIENTIFIC METHOD

Make Observations Students should make observations during their experimental procedure.

Form a Hypothesis Procedure step 3 asks students to form a hypothesis based on their initial observations.

Test the Hypothesis Procedure steps 4–11 guide students in designing and carrying out an experiment that tests their hypothesis.

Analyze the Results Analysis question 3 asks students to analyze their results.

Draw Conclusions Conclusions question 1 asks students to draw conclusions from their data.

MATERIALS

Instead of paper clips, students could use flat toothpicks to make their sensitivity testers.

SAFETY CAUTIONS

- Discuss the safety symbol with students.
- Caution students not to press hard with the sensitivity testers, but to use a very light touch.
- Each student should make his or her own tester to be used only by that student. Have students label their sensitivity testers with their names.

DISPOSAL

- Have students discard the testers after use.

TIPS AND TRICKS

Checkpoints

Make sure paper clips or toothpicks are securely fastened to the cardboard. The ends of the paper clips should be even so that they touch the skin at the same time. Students should bring the testers straight down so that the points touch the skin at the same time.

If students use the blindfold, make sure it is not too tight.

The test students are performing is referred to as the two-point discrimination test. Using this test, various areas of the body have been mapped for their relative sensitivity. Students may achieve clearer results if they select body areas with widely different sensitivities, rather than body areas that are very similar.

Body area	Two-point discrimination test values	Body area	Two-point discrimination test values
Finger	2–3 mm	Forehead	35 mm
Upper lip	4–5 mm	Forearm	35 mm
Cheek	6 mm	Neck	36 mm
Nose	7 mm	Upper arm	39 mm
Palm	10 mm	Shoulder	41 mm
Foot	20 mm	Thigh	42 mm
Belly	30 mm	Calf	45 mm

Sample Procedure

Unbend the paper clips and place two on each of six pieces of cardboard so that the paper clips lay flat and the straightened tips extend over the edge of the cardboard. Measure the distances between each pair of paper clips. Possible distances are 2 mm, 5 mm, 10 mm, 20 mm, 30 mm, and 40 mm. Carefully tape the paper clips into place. Measure again and make any necessary adjustments. Tape one paper clip to the seventh piece of cardboard.

Blindfold the subject, or have the subject keep the eyes closed during testing.

In random order, touch each of the seven testers to the body area being tested. Note if the subject detects one or two stimuli. Record the subject's response in a data table. Do additional trials if time permits.

Repeat the test on a different body area and record the results.

Inquiry Lab

DESIGN YOUR OWN

Distribution of Touch Receptors

In this lab, you will design and conduct an experiment to compare the distribution of touch receptors in the skin among different parts of the body.

OBJECTIVES

Develop a hypothesis to compare the sensitivities of different areas of the body to touch stimuli.

Design and **conduct** an experiment to test your hypothesis.

Evaluate your results and recognize the need to reduce bias in experimentation.

POSSIBLE MATERIALS

- blindfold
- corrugated cardboard, 3 × 5 cm (7)
- metric ruler
- paper clips (13)
- tape

Finding Out More Information

Skin, the largest organ of the human body, is sensitive to touch, pain, heat, and cold. Tactile sensation, or touch, relies on different types of receptors. One type of receptor is located deep in the dermis, the thick, inner layer of the skin. This receptor responds to strong pressure. Another type is located just below the epidermis, the outermost layer of the skin. This type of receptor responds to light touch. Touch receptors are located throughout your skin over your entire body. However, some areas of your skin have more touch receptors per square centimeter than do other areas.

If the touch receptors in the skin are relatively sparse, two stimuli applied to the skin will stimulate only one touch receptor and, thus, be perceived as one stimulus. If the receptors are spaced closely, two stimuli applied to the skin will stimulate two receptors and, thus, be perceived as two stimuli.

1. Which areas of the skin are likely to be more sensitive than others, that is, have more touch receptors?

   Answers will vary. Students may suggest that areas that are more important for gathering tactile information from the environment are likely to be more sensitive (have more receptors). Such areas would include the fingertips, palms, and face. Areas that need protection tend to be moderately sensitive and include the neck and abdomen. Areas that are less sensitive would include the back, shoulder, and legs.

Procedure

FORMING A HYPOTHESIS

Based on what you have learned, form a hypothesis about which areas of the skin are more sensitive (have more touch receptors) than others.

1. How can you determine the sensitivity of a particular area of the skin?

   Answers will vary. Based on the information given, students may suggest that varying the distance between two stimuli should give some indication of how sensitive a particular area is. The response of the test subject is recorded as to whether one or two stimuli are perceived.

2. How can you compare the relative sensitivities of different areas of the skin?

   Answers will vary. Based on the information given, students may suggest testing one area first by varying the distance between two stimuli, then testing another area in the same way. The test subject's responses to the varying distances between stimuli could then be compared to give an idea of relative sensitivity.

3. Write your hypothesis. A possible hypothesis might be "The skin on the calf is [more/less] sensitive than the skin on the palm, and the skin on the palm is [more/less] sensitive than the skin on the forearm.

   The skin on the cheek is more sensitive than the skin on the palm, and the skin on the palm is more sensitive than the skin on the forearm.

COMING UP WITH A PLAN

Plan and conduct an experiment to compare how sensitive the skin is on various parts of the body.

4. Write out a procedure for your experiment on a separate sheet of paper. As you plan the procedure, make the following decisions.
   - Decide which areas of the body you will test. Areas to consider include the fingers, calf, palm, forearm, upper arm, and neck.
   - Decide how to construct a device (or devices) for stimulating the skin, using the materials provided or other materials that you choose.
   - Decide on the number of trials you will run for each area of the body.

- Be sure to include a control that prevents the test subject from anticipating two stimuli and, therefore, guessing that two stimuli are present even when both are not felt. This type of response is referred to as bias because the subject's response may be based on the subject's expectation, rather than on the subject's observation. The possibility of bias exists when a person's subjective evaluation is required in an experiment. Bias can be difficult, but not impossible, to control.

5. Decide what safety procedures are necessary. Add them to your written procedure.

6. Using graph paper or a computer, construct tables to organize your data. Be sure that your data tables contain the appropriate information for the procedure you are following.

7. Have your teacher approve your plan.

PERFORMING THE EXPERIMENT

8. Implement your plan, using the equipment and safety procedures that you selected.

9. Record your data in your tables. If necessary, revise your tables to include variables that you did not think of while planning your experiment.

10. At the end of the experiment, pool the class data and determine the relative sensitivity of different areas of the body.

11. When you have finished, clean and store your equipment. Recycle or dispose of all materials as instructed by your teacher.

Analysis

SAMPLE TABLE

Distance between stimuli	Number of stimuli perceived					
	Calf		Palm		Forearm	
	Subject 1	Subject 2	Subject 1	Subject 2	Subject 1	Subject 2
1 stimulus						
2 mm						
5 mm	2	2				
10 mm			2	2		
20 mm						
30 mm					2	
40 mm						2

1. **Summarizing Data** What was the minimum distance between stimuli at which the test subject could consistently sense them as two points on the body parts you tested?

   Answers will vary but should be approximately 45 mm for the calf, 10 mm for the palm, and 35 mm for the forearm.

2. **Identifying/Recognizing Patterns** Relate your results to the number of skin receptors.

   The greater number of correct responses for a given body area, the larger the number of skin receptors in that area.

3. **Analyzing Data** Were there any differences between the data obtained for you and your partner? What could account for this?

   There is likely to be some variation in data between subjects due to individual variation and subjectivity, but the general pattern of sensitivity differences among body areas is likely to be consistent.

Conclusions

1. **Drawing Conclusions** Based on your data, rank the areas of the body that you tested from most to least sensitive.

   Most sensitive is the palm, and then the forearm, followed by the calf.

2. **Evaluating Methods** What was your control to minimize bias, that is, to keep the subject from guessing the number of stimuli being tested?

   One of the test stimuli should have had only one stimulus point.

3. **Evaluating Methods** Besides the control in question 1, what other type of controls did you use, or could have used to minimize bias?

   The presentation of the different test stimuli should be randomized with the control to minimize guessing and bias. Also, more than one trial could be run for each body part.

4. Applying Conclusions Describe a situation in which expectations could produce data that are in error.

Answers will vary. A possible answer is when a patient believes that a medication relieves symptoms, even when a placebo has been administered.

5. Applying Conclusions What kinds of results would you expect if you were to test other body parts? Examples include the finger, lip, nose, foot, forehead, belly, upper arm, neck, shoulder and thigh. Give a reason for your answer.

Answers will vary. Students should be able to generalize that the finger, lip, nose, and foot will probably be more sensitive than the forehead, belly, neck, and upper arm, which in turn, are generally more sensitive than the shoulder and thigh. Students who actually tested any of these areas should share their results with the class. Students should relate relative sensitivity to adaptive value. Body areas that come into contact with the environment first and gather information about the environment tend to be be most sensitive. Areas that don't gather as much information but still need protection tend to be moderately sensitive. Areas that don't gather as much information or need as much protection tend to be least sensitive.

Answer Key

Directed Reading

SECTION: BODY ORGANIZATION

1. connective
2. muscle
3. epithelial
4. nervous
5. connective
6. Smooth muscle is involuntary muscle found in visceral organs and walls of blood vessels. Skeletal muscle is voluntary muscle that moves bones in the trunk and limbs.
7. Embryonic stem cells are early, undifferentiated cells that give rise to all types of cells of the developing body. They divide indefinitely.
8. Tissues are groups of similar cells that perform a common function. Organs are made of combinations of two or more tissues and belong to at least one organ system.
9. The thoracic cavity encases the heart and lungs. The cranial cavity encases the brain. The abdominal cavity encases the digestive organs. The spinal cavity encases the spinal cord.
10. regulating body temperature, adjusting metabolism, detecting and responding to environmental stimuli, and maintaining water and mineral balances

SECTION: SKELETAL SYSTEM

1. The axial skeleton includes bones of the skull, spine, ribs, and sternum. All other bones, including those of the arms, legs, shoulders, and pelvis, make up the appendicular skeleton.
2. Bone marrow is a soft tissue that fills some cavities in spongy bone and that starts the production of blood cells. Periosteum is a tough membrane that covers bone.
3. Haversian canals are hollow channels in bone tissue that contain blood vessels that supply nutrients to osteocytes.
4. Osteoporosis is caused by the loss of bone density as people age.
5. Joints are junctions between bones. Ligaments are strong bands of connective tissue that hold the bones of a joint together.
6. Immovable joints permit little or no movement of the bones they join. Slightly moveable joints permit limited movement.
7. b
8. c
9. a

SECTION: MUSCULAR SYSTEM

1. bones
2. tendons
3. flexor
4. extensor
5. the ability to contract, the ability to stretch, and the ability to respond to stimuli
6. Myofibrils are small, cylindrical structures that make up muscle fibers. Sarcomeres, the functional units of muscle contraction, are the lengthwise sections of a myofibril.
7. b
8. e
9. a
10. c
11. d

SECTION: SKIN, HAIR, AND NAILS

1. epidermis
2. keratin
3. replaced
4. melanin
5. dermis
6. hair follicles
7. Blood vessels in the dermis dilate to release heat from the body and constrict to conserve body heat. Releasing sweat produced by sweat glands cools the body.
8. Subcutaneous tissue acts as a shock absorber, provides insulation to conserve body heat, stores energy, and anchors skin to organs.
9. sebum
10. oil

11. Carcinomas are skin cancers that originate in cells of the epidermis that do not produce pigments. Malignant melanomas are cancers that arise from pigment-producing cells and spread very quickly.
12. Skin cancer can result from genetic mutations caused by overexposure to UV radiation.

Active Reading

SECTION: BODY ORGANIZATION

1. Connective tissue cells in bone are densely packed, while those found in blood are spaced apart from each other.
2. The actions of voluntary muscle can be consciously controlled, while those of involuntary muscle cannot be consciously controlled.
3. smooth muscle
4. nerve tissue
5. skeletal muscle
6. epithelial tissue
7. connective tissue
8. cardiac muscle
9. epithelial tissue
10. connective tissue
11. epithelial tissue
12. nervous tissue
13. cardiac muscle
14. d

SECTION: SKELETAL SYSTEM

1. red bone marrow
2. mostly of fat
3. nutrients
4. bone marrow
5. spongy bone
6. compact bone
7. periosteum
8. This dense connective tissue forms the hard outer shell of a bone.
9. This loosely structured network of separated connective tissue forms a bone's porous inner core.
10. b

SECTION: MUSCULAR SYSTEM

1. The connective tissue holds muscle cells together and provides elasticity.
2. Actin and myosin are both protein filaments that enable muscles to contract.
3. They trigger a specific response by muscle tissue.
4. Z line
5. myofibril
6. myosin
7. actin
8. sarcomere
9. thin protein filaments found in muscle tissue that enable muscles to contract
10. small cylindrical structures that form a muscle fiber
11. thick protein filaments found in muscle tissue that enable muscles to contract
12. area between two Z lines, which contains overlapping protein filaments that interact with one another
13. center of each light-colored band of a myofibril that anchors actin filaments
14. d

SECTION: SKIN, HAIR, AND NAILS

1. acne; a chronic inflammatory condition that involves the skin's oil-producing glands
2. sebum; an oily secretion that lubricates the skin
3. pores
4. a

Vocabulary Review

1. e
2. a
3. d
4. b
5. c
6. axial skeleton
7. appendicular skeleton
8. marrow
9. periosteum
10. Haversian canals
11. osteocytes
12. osteoporosis
13. joint
14. ligaments
15. tendons
16. flexor
17. extensor
18. actin
19. myosin
20. myofibrils
21. sarcomere
22. c
23. a

24. f
25. b
26. e
27. g
28. d

Science Skills

INTERPRETING GRAPHICS

1. A—myosin; B—actin. The thicker myosin filaments have long, fingerlike projections with enlarged heads at one end. These heads attach to the binding sites on the actin filaments. Actin filaments are thin filaments that have sites to which myosin filaments can bind.
2. The two protein filaments slide past each other during muscle contraction.
3. Contraction begins as actin and myosin overlap. A myosin head attaches to a binding site on an actin filament. The myosin head then rotates, causing the actin filament to "slide" against the myosin filament. The sarcomere becomes shorter as the Z lines are pulled closer together and the muscle contracts.
4. ATP is needed for myosin to detach from actin.

5. O
6. I
7. G
8. C
9. D
10. F
11. L
12. J
13. Q
14. M
15. E
16. A
17. K
18. N
19. H
20. B
21. P
22. The skeleton provides structure and support, gives shape to the body, protects internal organs, and provides a framework for muscles.
23. The axial skeleton makes up the axis or center of the skeleton and includes the skull, spine, ribs, and sternum. The appendicular skeleton includes the remaining bones.

Concept Mapping

1. organ systems
2. organs
3. connective tissue or epithelial tissue or nervous tissue
4. epithelial tissue or connective tissue or nervous tissue
5. pancreas
6. nervous tissue or connective tissue or epithelial tissue
7. muscular system
8. skeletal muscle or cardiac muscle
9. cardiac muscle or skeletal muscle
10. appendicular skeleton or axial skeleton
11. axial skeleton or appendicular skeleton
12. hair or nails or skin
13. skin or hair or nails
14. nails or skin or hair

Critical Thinking

1. a
2. c
3. e
4. b
5. d
6. d
7. a
8. e
9. b
10. c
11. d
12. a
13. c
14. b
15. e, d
16. g, b
17. k, m
18. n, l
19. f, i
20. h, j
21. a, c
22. d
23. b
24. c
25. a

Test Prep Pretest

1. b
2. d
3. d
4. c
5. d
6. e
7. h
8. c
9. g
10. f
11. b
12. d
13. a
14. urinary bladder, urethra
15. exercise, minerals
16. myofibrils
17. aerobic, anaerobic
18. melanin
19. keratin
20. blood vessels
21. epidermis

22. sebum
23. Immovable joints permit little or no movement of the bones they join. The sutures that join the cranial bones of the skull are immovable joints. Slightly movable joints are joints that permit limited movement of the bones they join. Vertebrae in the spine are joined by slightly movable joints. Freely movable joints are joints that permit the greatest degree of movement. The hinge joints in the elbows and knees, the ball-and-socket joints of the shoulders and hips, and the saddle joints of the thumbs are all freely movable joints.
24. In a relaxed muscle fiber, the ends of the myosin and actin filaments in each sarcomere barely overlap. When the muscle fiber contracts, adjacent myosin and actin filaments slide along one another so that they overlap a great deal, shortening each sarcomere.
25. The epidermis, the outer layer of the skin, is made of a thin layer of dead cells. The dermis, the functional layer of skin beneath the epidermis, contains nerves, blood vessels, and lymph vessels. Subcutaneous tissue is a layer of fat-rich cells just beneath the dermis.

Quiz

SECTION: BODY ORGANIZATION

1. c	6. d
2. e	7. b
3. b	8. d
4. a	9. c
5. d	10. a

SECTION: SKELETAL SYSTEM

1. c	6. c
2. a	7. c
3. d	8. a
4. e	9. d
5. b	10. b

SECTION: MUSCULAR SYSTEM

1. c	6. b
2. e	7. c
3. d	8. c
4. a	9. d
5. b	10. a

SECTION: SKIN, HAIR, AND NAILS

1. b	6. d
2. c	7. b
3. a	8. c
4. e	9. d
5. d	10. a

Chapter Test (General)

1. c	11. c
2. c	12. c
3. d	13. a
4. c	14. b
5. d	15. d
6. a	16. a
7. b	17. c
8. b	18. b
9. d	19. c
10. d	20. a

Chapter Test (Advanced)

1. b
2. b
3. b
4. a
5. b
6. d
7. d
8. endothermy
9. axial skeleton
10. flexors
11. oxygen, oxygen
12. hair follicles
13. embryonic stem cells
14. e
15. b
16. g
17. d
18. c
19. f
20. a
21. Myosin and actin filaments lie parallel along the length of a myofibril in units called sarcomeres. The myosin heads touch the adjacent actin filaments. When a muscle fiber is stimulated, the myosin heads attach to the actin filaments. The myosin heads bend inward, pulling the actin filaments. As the filaments slide against one another, Z lines move closer together, shortening the sarcomere. The entire muscle fiber contracts.

22. The outermost layer of the skin is the epidermis. This layer is responsible for protection from the environment. Accessory structures, such as hair and nails, are derived from cells of the epidermis.

23. Blood vessels within the periosteum supply nutrients to bone tissue. Within each Haversian canal, smaller blood vessels carry nutrients to individual osteocytes. Because the Haversian canals extend down the length of a bone, nutrients and waste products can be transported to and from osteocytes anywhere within the bone.

24. Structures in the dermis help regulate body temperature. Blood vessels in the dermis will dilate or constrict in order to release or conserve body heat, respectively. Sweat glands produce sweat, which evaporates from the surface of the skin, releasing excess body heat.

25. Carcinomas and malignant melanomas both originate in the epidermis. Avoiding overexposure to either natural or artificial UV radiation can help prevent the development of skin cancer. Regular self-examination of moles for changes in shape, size, and color is also helpful.

Lesson Plan

Section: Body Organization

Pacing

Regular Schedule:	**with lab(s):** N/A	**without lab(s):** 3 days
Block Schedule:	**with lab(s):** N/A	**without lab(s):** 1 1/2 days

Objectives

1. Identify four levels of structural organization within the human body.
2. Analyze the four kinds of body tissue.
3. List the body's major organ systems.
4. Evaluate the importance of endothermy in maintaining homeostasis.

National Science Education Standards Covered

UNIFYING CONCEPTS AND PROCESSES

UCP1: Systems, order, and organization

UCP5: Form and function

SCIENCE AS INQUIRY

SI1: Abilities necessary to do scientific inquiry

SI2: Understandings about scientific inquiry

LIFE SCIENCE: MATTER, ENERGY, AND ORGANIZATION IN LIVING SYSTEMS

LSMat4: The complexity and organization of organisms accommodates the need for obtaining, transforming, transporting, releasing, and eliminating the matter and energy used to sustain the organism.

LSMat6: As matter and energy flow through different levels of organization of living systems—cells, organs, communities—and between living systems and the physical environment, chemical elements are recombined in different ways.

PHYSICAL SCIENCE

PS6: Interactions of energy and matter

KEY
SE = Student Edition
TE = Teacher Edition
CRF = Chapter Resource File

Block 1

CHAPTER OPENER *(45 minutes)*

_ **Quick Review,** SE. Students answer questions covered in previous sections of the textbook as preparation for the chapter content. **(GENERAL)**

_ **Reading Activity,** SE. Students draw and label a diagram of an idealized mollusk. **(GENERAL)**

_ **Using the Figure,** TE. Students answer questions about the chapter opener photograph. **(GENERAL)**

_ **Opening Activity**, Doing Simple Tasks, TE. Students identify which body systems are used to perform a simple task, such as opening a jar or tuning a radio. **(BASIC)**

Block 2

FOCUS *(5 minutes)*

_ **Bellringer Transparency.** Use this transparency as students enter the classroom and find their seats. **(GENERAL)**

MOTIVATE *(10 minutes)*

_ **Discussion/Question**, TE. Students discuss the activities of the stomach and the different types of tissue found in the stomach. **(GENERAL)**

TEACH *(30 minutes)*

_ **Teaching Transparency, Section Outline.** Use this transparency to give students a framework for the information in this section. **(GENERAL)**

_ **Directed Reading Worksheet, Body Organization, CRF.** Students complete the exercises in this worksheet to help them understand the material as they read the section. **(BASIC)**

_ **Teaching Transparency, Human Body Tissues.** Use this transparency to review the epithelial tissue, nervous tissue, connective tissue, and muscle tissue in the human body. **(GENERAL)**

_ **Inclusion Strategies**, TE. Students design a class chart of the four types of tissue found in the body. Students can also design a chart of the types of muscle tissue. **(BASIC)**

HOMEWORK

_ **Active Reading Worksheet, Body Organization, CRF.** Students read a passage related to the section topic and answer questions. **(GENERAL)**

Block 3

TEACH *(30 minutes)*

_ **Teaching Transparency, Major Organ Systems of the Human Body.** Use this transparency to review the major structures and functions of the major organ systems found in the human body. **(GENERAL)**

_ **Activity**, Organizational Hierarchy, TE. Students make a graphic organizer to demonstrate that simpler structures in the body are components of more-complex structures. **(BASIC)**

_ **Teaching Transparency, Cavities of the Human Body.** Use this transparency to point out that the human body contains four large fluid-filled cavities, which house and protect the major internal organs. **(GENERAL)**

_ **Teaching Transparency, Inside the Human Coelom.** Use this transparency to illustrate the two compartments in the human coelom. Review the evolutionary and developmental history of the coelom. Ask students how food passes through the thoracic cavity into the stomach, which is in the abdominal cavity. **(GENERAL)**

CLOSE *(15 minutes)*

_ **Reteaching,** TE. Use a situation familiar to students to help them understand the levels of organization in the body. For example, a house is part of a city, which is part of a county, which is part of a state, which is part of the United States. **(BASIC)**

_ **Quiz,** TE. Students answer questions that review the section material. **(GENERAL)**

HOMEWORK

_ **Section Review,** SE. Assign questions 1–6 for review, homework, or quiz. **(GENERAL)**

_ **Quiz, CRF.** This quiz consists of ten multiple choice and matching questions that review the section's main concepts. **(BASIC) Also in Spanish.**

Other Resource Options

_ **Reading Skill Builder**, Interactive Reading, TE. Students listen to the chapter on the *Holt Biology* Guided Audio CD Program. **(BASIC)**

_ **Teaching Tip**, Tissue and Organ Transplants, TE. Students list body parts that have been transplanted in humans and identify them as tissues or organs. **(GENERAL)**

_ **Internet Connect.** Students can research Internet sources about Organ Systems with SciLinks Code HX4131.

_ **go.hrw.com.** For worksheets, videos, and other teaching aids related to this chapter, visit the HRW Web site and type in the keyword HX4 BDY.

_ **CNN Student News.** Find the latest news, lesson plans, and activities related to important scientific events at **cnnstudentnews.com**.

Lesson Plan

Section: Skeletal System

Pacing

Regular Schedule:	**with lab(s):** 3 days	**without lab(s):** 2 days
Block Schedule:	**with lab(s):** 1 1/2 days	**without lab(s):** 1 day

Objectives

1. Distinguish between the axial skeleton and the appendicular skeleton.
2. Analyze the structure of bone.
3. Summarize the process of bone development.
4. List two ways to prevent osteoporosis.
5. Identify the three main classes of joints.

National Science Education Standards Covered

UNIFYING CONCEPTS AND PROCESSES

UCP1: Systems, order, and organization

UCP5: Form and function

SCIENCE AS INQUIRY

SI1: Abilities necessary to do scientific inquiry

SI2: Understandings about scientific inquiry

LIFE SCIENCE: MATTER, ENERGY, AND ORGANIZATION IN LIVING SYSTEMS

LSMat4: The complexity and organization of organisms accommodates the need for obtaining, transforming, transporting, releasing, and eliminating the matter and energy used to sustain the organism.

LSMat6: As matter and energy flow through different levels of organization of living systems—cells, organs, communities—and between living systems and the physical environment, chemical elements are recombined in different ways.

PHYSICAL SCIENCE

PS6: Interactions of energy and matter

KEY
SE = Student Edition
CRF = Chapter Resource File
TE = Teacher Edition

Block 4

FOCUS *(5 minutes)*

_ **Bellringer Transparency.** Use this transparency as students enter the classroom and find their seats. **(GENERAL)**

MOTIVATE *(10 minutes)*

_ **Discussion/Question**, TE. Students discuss what they already know about joints. Given the names of the types of joints, students provide an example of each type and describe the movement for which each type is adapted. **(GENERAL)**

TEACH *(30 minutes)*

_ **Teaching Transparency, Section Outline.** Use this transparency to give students a framework for the information in this section. **(GENERAL)**

_ **Directed Reading Worksheet, Skeletal System, CRF.** Students complete the exercises in this worksheet to help them understand the material as they read the section. **(BASIC)**

_ **Teaching Transparency, Human Skeleton.** Use this transparency to discuss the major bones that make up the human skeleton. Point out the axial skeleton, the appendicular skeleton, and the major skeletal bones. **(GENERAL)**

_ **Teaching Transparency, Structure of Bone Tissue.** Use this transparency to illustrate the structure of bone tissue. Review the terms *spongy bone, compact bone,* and *bone marrow.* **(GENERAL)**

_ **Teaching Transparency, Compact Bone.** Use this transparency to point out the concentric rings of bone surrounding Haversian canals in compact bone. **(GENERAL)**

HOMEWORK

_ **Inclusion Strategies**, TE. Students research osteoporosis and make a taped or live public service announcement or brochure to share their findings.

_ **Active Reading Worksheet, Skeletal System, CRF.** Students read a passage related to the section topic and answer questions. **(GENERAL)**

Block 5

TEACH *(30 minutes)*

_ **Group Activity,** Spinal Flexibility, TE. Students make a model of the vertebral column using thread spools and a long shoelace. **(BASIC)**

- **Demonstration,** TE. Students compare the flexibility of a chicken bone that has been cooked, cleaned, and soaked overnight in vinegar (to remove much of the calcium) with the flexibility of a cooked, clean bone that has not been soaked. Relate these ideas to what happens to bone because of osteoporosis. **(GENERAL)**
- **Teaching Transparency, Effects of Osteoporosis.** Use this transparency to discuss the effects of osteoporosis on bones. Ask students which people are at the most risk of getting osteoporosis. Ask students to list ways to prevent osteoporosis. **(GENERAL)**
- **Teaching Transparency, The Human Knee.** Use this transparency to discuss the knee as an example of a freely movable joint. Point out the parts of the knee. **(GENERAL)**

CLOSE *(15 minutes)*

- **Reteaching,** TE. Students examine prepared slides of cartilage and bone and explain how the structure of cartilage and the structure of bone are related to the function each performs in the body. **(BASIC)**
- **Quiz,** TE. Students answer questions that review the section material. **(GENERAL)**

HOMEWORK

- **Section Review,** SE. Assign questions 1–7 for review, homework, or quiz. **(GENERAL)**
- **Quiz, CRF.** This quiz consists of ten multiple choice and matching questions that review the section's main concepts. **(BASIC) Also in Spanish.**

Optional Block

LAB *(45 minutes)*

- **Quick Lab, Comparing Skeletal Joints, CRF.** Students explore the types of skeletal joints found in the body by observing an example of each type of joint and surveying the other joints in the body. **(BASIC)**

Other Resource Options

- **Alternative Assessment,** TE. Students make models of joints and bone cross sections using readily available materials. **(GENERAL)**
- **Internet Connect.** Students can research Internet sources about Joint Disorders with SciLinks Code HX4107.
- **go.hrw.com.** For worksheets, videos, and other teaching aids related to this chapter, visit the HRW Web site and type in the keyword HX4 BDY.
- **CNN Student News.** Find the latest news, lesson plans, and activities related to important scientific events at **cnnstudentnews.com**.

Lesson Plan

Section: Muscular System

Pacing

Regular Schedule:	**with lab(s):** N/A	**without lab(s):** 2 days
Block Schedule:	**with lab(s):** N/A	**without lab(s):** 1 day

Objectives

1. Describe the action of muscle pairs in moving the body.
2. Relate the structure of a skeletal muscle to the muscle's ability to contract.
3. Describe how energy is supplied to muscles for contraction.

National Science Education Standards Covered

UNIFYING CONCEPTS AND PROCESSES

UCP1: Systems, order, and organization

UCP5: Form and function

SCIENCE AS INQUIRY

SI1: Abilities necessary to do scientific inquiry

SI2: Understandings about scientific inquiry

LIFE SCIENCE: MATTER, ENERGY, AND ORGANIZATION IN LIVING SYSTEMS

LSMat4: The complexity and organization of organisms accommodates the need for obtaining, transforming, transporting, releasing, and eliminating the matter and energy used to sustain the organism.

PHYSICAL SCIENCE

PS6: Interactions of energy and matter

KEY
SE = Student Edition **TE** = Teacher Edition
CRF = Chapter Resource File

Block 6

FOCUS *(5 minutes)*

_ **Bellringer Transparency.** Use this transparency as students enter the classroom and find their seats. **(GENERAL)**

MOTIVATE *(5 minutes)*

_ **Demonstration**, TE. Have a volunteer demonstrate how the biceps and triceps work. **(GENERAL)**

TEACH *(35 minutes)*

_ **Teaching Transparency, Section Outline.** Use this transparency to give students a framework for the information in this section. **(GENERAL)**

_ **Teaching Transparency, Opposing Muscles in the Arm.** Use this transparency to discuss how pairs of opposing muscles work together to move bones at joints. **(GENERAL)**

_ **Teaching Transparency, Structure of Skeletal Muscle.** Use this transparency to discuss the structures that make up skeletal muscle. Review the terms *myofibril, sarcomere, Z line, actin filament,* and *myosin filament.* Point out the levels of organization shown in the figure. **(GENERAL)**

_ **Demonstration**, TE. Students use diagrams to compare the muscles of insects and vertebrates. **(GENERAL)**

_ **Teaching Transparency, Contraction of a Muscle.** Use this transparency when describing the events underlying muscle contraction: attachment of myosin heads to actin, bending of myosin heads, release of bonds between myosin and actin, and recocking of myosin heads for the next cycle. **(GENERAL)**

HOMEWORK

_ **Directed Reading Worksheet, Muscular System, CRF.** Students complete the exercises in this worksheet to help them understand the material as they read the section. **(BASIC)**

_ **Active Reading Worksheet, Muscular System, CRF.** Students read a passage related to the section topic and answer questions. **(GENERAL)**

Block 7

TEACH *(30 minutes)*

_ **Teaching Tip**, TE. Students research muscle contraction and draw a diagram of a sarcomere before and during contraction. **(GENERAL)**

_ **Teaching Transparency, Interaction of Muscle Protein Filaments.** Use this transparency to discuss how myosin and actin interact. Point out that the myosin heads attach to the binding sites on actin filaments and then rotate, causing myosin to move relative to actin. **(GENERAL)**

_ **Integrating Physics and Chemistry**, TE. Students compare human body joints with simple machines, such as levers, planes, and pulleys.

_ **Activity**, TE. Students do a finger exercise to show that the tendons in the middle finger and the ring finger are linked.

CLOSE *(15 minutes)*

- **Reteaching,** TE. Students create a flip book of 20 or more pages showing the mechanics of muscle contraction. **(BASIC)**
- **Quiz,** TE. Students answer questions that review the section material. **(GENERAL)**

HOMEWORK

- **Alternative Assessment,** TE. Students draw a diagram that illustrates the role of ATP in muscle contraction and that shows each step in the muscle contraction process. **(GENERAL)**
- **Section Review,** SE. Assign questions 1–5 for review, homework, or quiz. **(GENERAL)**
- **Quiz, CRF.** This quiz consists of ten multiple choice and matching questions that review the section's main concepts. **(BASIC) Also in Spanish.**

Other Resource Options

- **Internet Connect.** Students can research Internet sources about Muscle Structure with SciLinks Code HX4126.
- **Internet Connect.** Students can research Internet sources about Muscle Contraction with SciLinks Code HX4087.
- **go.hrw.com.** For worksheets, videos, and other teaching aids related to this chapter, visit the HRW Web site and type in the keyword HX4 BDY.
- **CNN Student News.** Find the latest news, lesson plans, and activities related to important scientific events at **cnnstudentnews.com**.

Lesson Plan

Section: Skin, Hair, and Nails

Pacing

Regular Schedule:	**with lab(s):** 3 days	**without lab(s):** 2 days
Block Schedule:	**with lab(s):** 1 1/2 days	**without lab(s):** 1 day

Objectives

1. Analyze the structure and function of the epidermis.
2. Describe how the dermis helps the body maintain homeostasis.
3. Summarize how hair and nails are formed.
4. Identify various types of skin disorders.

National Science Education Standards Covered

UNIFYING CONCEPTS AND PROCESSES

UCP1: Systems, order, and organization

UCP5: Form and function

SCIENCE AS INQUIRY

SI1: Abilities necessary to do scientific inquiry

SI2: Understandings about scientific inquiry

LIFE SCIENCE: MATTER, ENERGY, AND ORGANIZATION IN LIVING SYSTEMS

LSMat4: The complexity and organization of organisms accommodates the need for obtaining, transforming, transporting, releasing, and eliminating the matter and energy used to sustain the organism.

LSMat6: As matter and energy flow through different levels of organization of living systems—cells, organs, communities—and between living systems and the physical environment, chemical elements are recombined in different ways.

PHYSICAL SCIENCE

PS6: Interactions of energy and matter

KEY
SE = Student Edition   **TE** = Teacher Edition
CRF = Chapter Resource File

Block 8

FOCUS *(5 minutes)*

_ **Bellringer Transparency.** Use this transparency as students enter the classroom and find their seats. **(GENERAL)**

MOTIVATE *(10 minutes)*

_ **Discussion**, TE. Ask students questions to find out what they know about ultraviolet light, suntanning, and skin cancer. **(GENERAL)**

TEACH *(30 minutes)*

_ **Teaching Transparency, Section Outline.** Use this transparency to give students a framework for the information in this section. **(GENERAL)**

_ **Directed Reading Worksheet, Skin, Hair, and Nails, CRF.** Students complete the exercises in this worksheet to help them understand the material as they read the section. **(BASIC)**

_ **Teaching Transparency, Structure of Skin.** Use this transparency to review the structures found in each layer of skin. Point out the hair follicles and shafts, oil glands, sweat glands, and sweat pores and emphasize which structures pass through both layers of skin. **(GENERAL)**

HOMEWORK

_ **Active Reading Worksheet, Skin, Hair, and Nails, CRF.** Students read a passage related to the section topic and answer questions. **(GENERAL)**

Block 9

TEACH *(25 minutes)*

_ **Teaching Tip,** Skin Layers, TE. Students make a graphic organizer to demonstrate the relationship between the skin's two primary layers and the subcutaneous tissue. **(GENERAL)**

_ **Skill Builder,** Writing, TE. Students research skin cancer using the Internet sites suggested under Other Resource Options Internet Connect. Then students write a paragraph on the risk factors and symptoms of two relatively common carninomas and identify the primary risk factor for nearly all types of skin cancer. **(ADVANCED)**

- **Teaching Tip**, Homeothermy, TE. Use the difference in appearance of raw egg white and cooked egg white to illustrate the effects of high temperature on proteins. **(BASIC)**

CLOSE *(20 minutes)*

- **Reteaching,** TE. Use rapid-fire questions to review the layers of the skin and the important structures in each layer. **(BASIC)**
- **Alternative Assessment,** TE. Students make a three-dimensional model of the skin using construction paper, tissue paper, yarn, glue, or other art materials. Ask students to show and explain their models to the class. **(GENERAL)**
- **Quiz,** TE. Students answer questions that review the section material. **(GENERAL)**

HOMEWORK

- **Section Review,** SE. Assign questions 1–6 for review, homework, or quiz. **(GENERAL)**
- **Quiz, CRF.** This quiz consists of ten multiple choice and matching questions that review the section's main concepts. **(BASIC) Also in Spanish.**
- **Modified Worksheet, One-Stop Planner.** This worksheet has been specially modified to reach struggling students. **(BASIC)**
- **Critical Thinking Worksheet, CRF.** Students answer analogy-based questions that review the section's main concepts and vocabulary. **(ADVANCED)**

Optional Block

LAB *(45 minutes)*

- **Inquiry Lab, Distribution of Touch Receptors, CRF.** Students design and conduct an experiment to compare the distribution of touch receptors in the skin among different parts of the body. **(GENERAL)**

Other Resource Options

- **Interactive Exploration,** Life Span and Lifestyle. Students use a CD-ROM simulation to explore how exercise, diet, smoking, and drinking alcohol affect life span. **(GENERAL)**
- **Datasheets for In-Text Labs, Life Span and Lifestyle, CRF.**
- **Science Skills Worksheet, CRF.** Students interpret a diagram of muscle contraction and label the bones on a diagram of the human skeleton. **(GENERAL)**
- **Exploration Lab,** Analyzing the Work of Muscles, SE. Students investigate how fatigue affects the amount of work that muscles can do. **(GENERAL)**
- **Datasheets for In-Text Labs, Analyzing the Work of Muscles, CRF.**
- **Supplemental Reading, Microbe Hunters, One-Stop Planner.** Students read the book and answer questions. **(ADVANCED)**

- **Internet Connect.** Students can research Internet sources about Forensic Analysis with SciLinks Code HX4087.
- **Internet Connect.** Students can research Internet sources about Skin Cancer with SciLinks Code HX4165.
- **go.hrw.com.** For worksheets, videos, and other teaching aids related to this chapter, visit the HRW Web site and type in the keyword HX4 BDY.
- **CNN Science in the News, Video Segment 30 Tanning Effects.** This video segment is accompanied by a **Critical Thinking Worksheet**.
- **CNN Student News.** Find the latest news, lesson plans, and activities related to important scientific events at **cnnstudentnews.com**.

Lesson Plan

End-of-Chapter Review and Assessment

Pacing

Regular Schedule: 2 days

Block Schedule: 1 day

KEY	
SE = Student Edition	TE = Teacher Edition
CRF = Chapter Resource File	

Block 10

REVIEW *(45 minutes)*

_ **Study Zone,** SE. Use the Study Zone to review the Key Concepts and Key Terms of the chapter and prepare students for the Performance Zone questions. **(GENERAL)**

_ **Performance Zone,** SE. Assign questions to review the material for this chapter. Use the assignment guide to customize review for sections covered. **(GENERAL)**

_ **Teaching Transparency,** Concept Mapping. Use this transparency to review the concept map for this chapter. **(GENERAL)**

Block 11

ASSESSMENT *(45 minutes)*

_ **Chapter Test, Introduction to Body Structure, CRF.** This test contains 20 multiple choice and matching questions keyed to the chapter's objectives. **(GENERAL) Also in Spanish.**

_ **Chapter Test, Introduction to Body Structure, CRF.** This test contains 25 questions of various formats, each keyed to the chapter's objectives. **(ADVANCED)**

_ **Modified Chapter Test, One-Stop Planner.** This test has been specially modified to reach struggling students. **(BASIC)**

Other Resource Options

_ **Vocabulary Review Worksheet, CRF.** Use this worksheet to review the chapter vocabulary. **(GENERAL) Also in Spanish.**

_ **Test Prep Pretest, CRF.** Use this pretest to review the main content of the chapter. Each question is keyed to a section objective. **(GENERAL) Also in Spanish.**

_ **Test Item Listing for ExamView® Test Generator, CRF.** Use the Test Item Listing to identify questions to use in a customized homework, quiz, or test.

_ **ExamView® Test Generator, One-Stop Planner.** Create a customized homework, quiz, or test using the HRW Test Generator program.

Introduction to Body Structure

TRUE-FALSE

1. ____ The four basic types of tissue in the body are epithelial, muscle, nervous, and connective.
Answer: True Difficulty: I Section: 1 Objective: 2

2. ____ Cartilage is a type of connective tissue.
Answer: True Difficulty: I Section: 1 Objective: 2

3. ____ The smooth muscle that is found in the stomach walls is an example of voluntary muscle.
Answer: False Difficulty: I Section: 1 Objective: 2

4. ____ The three basic types of muscle are skeletal, smooth, and cardiac.
Answer: True Difficulty: I Section: 1 Objective: 2

5. ____ The excretory system filters metabolic wastes from the bloodstream and controls the concentration of body fluids.
Answer: True Difficulty: I Section: 1 Objective: 3

6. ____ Organs working together form an organ system.
Answer: True Difficulty: I Section: 1 Objective: 3

7. ____ Ectothermy is the primary factor that enables the human body to maintain homeostasis.
Answer: False Difficulty: I Section: 1 Objective: 4

8. ____ The hip attachment of the bones is called the pectoral girdle, and the shoulder attachment is called the pelvic girdle.
Answer: False Difficulty: I Section: 2 Objective: 1

9. ____ The majority of the bones of the skeleton are part of the axial skeleton.
Answer: False Difficulty: I Section: 2 Objective: 1

10. ____ Yellow bone marrow is contained in the shafts of the long bones.
Answer: True Difficulty: I Section: 2 Objective: 2

11. ____ The Haversian canals of long bones are filled with yellow marrow.
Answer: False Difficulty: I Section: 2 Objective: 3

12. ____ The chances of developing osteoporosis later in life are greatly reduced by a mineral-rich diet and regular exercise throughout life.
Answer: True Difficulty: I Section: 2 Objective: 4

13. ____ Osteoporosis is the painful inflammation of freely movable joints.
Answer: False Difficulty: I Section: 2 Objective: 4

14. ____ The bones of the knee are connected by semimovable joints.
Answer: False Difficulty: I Section: 2 Objective: 5

15. ____ The shoulder joint is an example of a ball-and socket joint.
Answer: True Difficulty: I Section: 2 Objective: 5

16. ____ Extensor muscles cause bones to bend at a joint, while flexors cause them to straighten.
Answer: False Difficulty: I Section: 3 Objective: 1

17. ____ Moving a muscle requires three sets of muscles working in opposition.
Answer: False Difficulty: I Section: 3 Objective: 1

18. ____ A sarcomere is composed of filaments called myofibrils.
Answer: False Difficulty: I Section: 3 Objective: 2

19. ____ Actin and myosin are proteins that enable muscles to contract.
Answer: True Difficulty: I Section: 3 Objective: 2

20. ____ When a muscle fiber contracts, the sarcomeres relax.
Answer: False Difficulty: I Section: 3 Objective: 2

21. ____ The total amount of force a muscle exerts during contraction depends on how many muscle fibers contract.
Answer: True Difficulty: I Section: 3 Objective: 2

22. ____ The binding of myosin heads to actin filaments during a muscle contraction causes the sarcomere to lengthen.
Answer: False Difficulty: I Section: 3 Objective: 2

23. ____ Aerobic exercise is done mainly to increase skeletal muscle size and strength.
Answer: False Difficulty: I Section: 3 Objective: 3

24. ____ Resistance exercises, such as chin-ups, use the most efficient pathway of producing ATP within the body.
Answer: False Difficulty: I Section: 3 Objective: 3

25. ____ The distribution of melanin in the epidermis of the skin determines the color of an individual.
Answer: True Difficulty: I Section: 4 Objective: 1

26. ____ The dermis is a dead layer of skin that is nonfunctional.
Answer: False Difficulty: I Section: 4 Objective: 2

27. ____ Each hair on your head grows indefinitely.
Answer: False Difficulty: I Section: 4 Objective: 3

28. ____ Nails are produced by specialized epidermal cells.
Answer: True Difficulty: I Section: 4 Objective: 3

29. ____ Sweat glands in the dermis help remove excess body heat.
Answer: True Difficulty: I Section: 4 Objective: 2

30. ____ Acne is caused by excessive sweating.
Answer: False Difficulty: I Section: 4 Objective: 4

31. ____ Most skin cancers result from mutations in the melanin-producing cells.
Answer: False Difficulty: I Section: 4 Objective: 4

MULTIPLE CHOICE

32. From the smallest functional units to the largest, the body is organized as follows:
a. cell, system, organ, tissue, body.
b. organ, cell, tissue, system, body.
c. system, organ, tissue, cell, body.
d. cell, tissue, organ, system, body.
Answer: D Difficulty: I Section: 1 Objective: 1

33. Tissue that is specialized to cover the inner and outer surfaces of the internal organs is called
a. epithelial tissue.
b. connective tissue.
c. muscle tissue.
d. nerve tissue.
Answer: A Difficulty: I Section: 1 Objective: 2

34. Tightly connected cells that are arranged in flat sheets are characteristic of
    a. epithelial tissue.
    b. connective tissue.
    c. muscle tissue.
    d. nerve tissue.

    Answer: A   Difficulty: I   Section: 1   Objective: 2

35. Blood, bone, and cartilage are examples of
    a. three different tissue types found in the body.
    b. connective tissue.
    c. epithelial tissue.
    d. organs of the body.

    Answer: B   Difficulty: I   Section: 1   Objective: 2

36. Connective tissue includes
    a. tendons.
    b. blood.
    c. fat.
    d. All of the above

    Answer: D   Difficulty: I   Section: 1   Objective: 2

37. The three types of muscle tissue are
    a. skeletal, smooth, and cardiac.
    b. skeletal, voluntary, and cardiac.
    c. smooth, cardiac, and involuntary.
    d. skeletal, cardiac, and ridged.

    Answer: A   Difficulty: I   Section: 1   Objective: 2

38. Smooth muscle
    a. can change the diameter of blood vessels.
    b. moves food through the digestive tract.
    c. is not under conscious control.
    d. All of the above

    Answer: D   Difficulty: I   Section: 1   Objective: 2

39. Smooth muscles can be found
    a. attached to the skeleton.
    b. in the wrist bones.
    c. at the knee joint.
    d. in internal organs.

    Answer: D   Difficulty: I   Section: 1   Objective: 2

40. Muscle tissue functions to move
    a. blood.
    b. food in the digestive tract.
    c. bones.
    d. All of the above

    Answer: D   Difficulty: I   Section: 1   Objective: 2

41. Organs that work together form
    a. connective tissues.
    b. tissue systems.
    c. organ systems.
    d. All of the above

    Answer: C   Difficulty: I   Section: 1   Objective: 3

42. The heart and the blood vessels are separate organs that form the
    a. skeletal system.
    b. circulatory system.
    c. reproductive system.
    d. digestive system.

    Answer: B   Difficulty: I   Section: 1   Objective: 3

43. Which of the following would likely occur if endothermy were disrupted?
    a. Body temperature could not be maintained.
    b. Strenuous physical activity would be difficult.
    c. Enzymes would be inactivated.
    d. All of the above

    Answer: D   Difficulty: I   Section: 1   Objective: 4

44. The heart and lungs are protected by the
    a. pectoral girdle.
    b. pelvic girdle.
    c. rib cage.
    d. periosteum.

    Answer: C   Difficulty: I   Section: 2   Objective: 1

45. Of the following, the structure that is *not* part of the axial skeleton is the
    a. backbone.
    b. pectoral girdle.
    c. rib cage.
    d. skull.

    Answer: B   Difficulty: I   Section: 2   Objective: 1

46. A person with a broken pelvic girdle would probably be unable to
    a. walk.
    b. turn his or her head.
    c. raise his or her arm.
    d. bend his or her wrist.

    Answer: A   Difficulty: I   Section: 2   Objective: 1

47. Yellow marrow
    a. provides internal support to spongy bone.
    b. produces red blood cells.
    c. is found only in lower vertebrates.
    d. consists mainly of fat that stores energy.

    Answer: D   Difficulty: I   Section: 2   Objective: 2

48. The type of bone that provides the greatest strength for support is
    a. spongy bone.
    b. chitinous bone.
    c. compact bone.
    d. marrow bone.

    Answer: C   Difficulty: I   Section: 2   Objective: 2

49. The periosteum is the tough exterior membrane that surrounds bones and that contains
    a. blood vessels.
    b. osteocytes.
    c. spongy bone.
    d. red bone marrow.

    Answer: A   Difficulty: I   Section: 2   Objective: 2

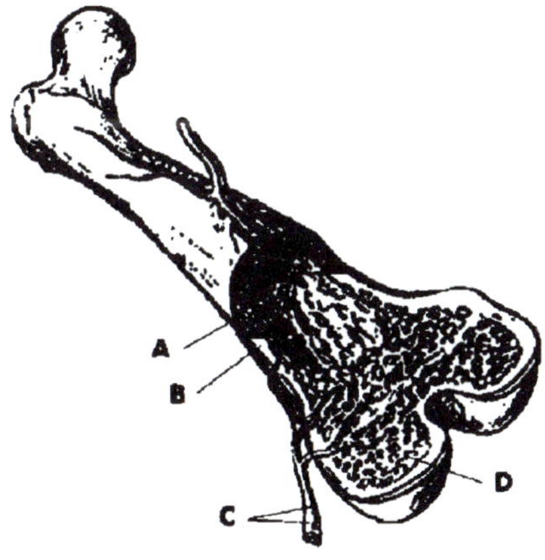

50. Refer to the illustration above. The compact bone is labeled
    a. A.
    b. B.
    c. C.
    d. D.

    Answer: B   Difficulty: II   Section: 2   Objective: 2

51. Refer to the illustration above. The material labeled A, which fills the center and spaces at ends and produces blood cells, is known as
    a. exocrine material.
    b. cartilage.
    c. bone marrow.
    d. spongy bone.

    Answer: C   Difficulty: II   Section: 2   Objective: 2

52. Refer to the illustration above. The structure labeled C is a
    a. nerve.
    b. blood vessel.
    c. muscle.
    d. ligament.

    Answer: B Difficulty: II Section: 2 Objective: 2

53. compact bone : periosteum ::
    a. periosteum : compact bone
    b. compact bone : spongy bone
    c. spongy bone : marrow
    d. marrow : compact bone

    Answer: D Difficulty: II Section: 2 Objective: 2

54. In an embryo, the skeleton is originally made of
    a. red and yellow marrow.
    b. calcium phosphate.
    c. cartilage.
    d. osteopores.

    Answer: C Difficulty: I Section: 2 Objective: 3

55. Bone cells that become embedded within the concentric layers of bone tissue are
    a. osteocytes.
    b. periosteal cells.
    c. red marrow cells.
    d. yellow marrow cells.

    Answer: A Difficulty: I Section: 2 Objective: 3

56. Osteocytes trapped within the spaces in the bone surrounding them
    a. are called marrow cells.
    b. are provided with food and oxygen by Haversian canals.
    c. receive nutrients directly from the cells of the surrounding cartilage.
    d. eventually become osteoblasts as the bone matures.

    Answer: B Difficulty: I Section: 2 Objective: 3

57. Bone loss may be slowed by
    a. calcium.
    b. regular exercise.
    c. a balanced diet.
    d. All of the above

    Answer: D Difficulty: I Section: 2 Objective: 4

58. Women are more susceptible than men to the effects of osteoporosis because
    a. their bones are smaller than those of men.
    b. they lose calcium during the child-bearing years.
    c. sex hormone production declines during menopause.
    d. All of the above

    Answer: D Difficulty: I Section: 2 Objective: 4

59. The loss of bone density that may occur in the later years of life is called
    a. menopause.
    b. bone replacement.
    c. bone fractures.
    d. osteoporosis.

    Answer: D Difficulty: I Section: 2 Objective: 4

60. The point where two or more bones meet is called a
    a. sprain.
    b. joint.
    c. point of intersection.
    d. growth region.

    Answer: B Difficulty: I Section: 2 Objective: 5

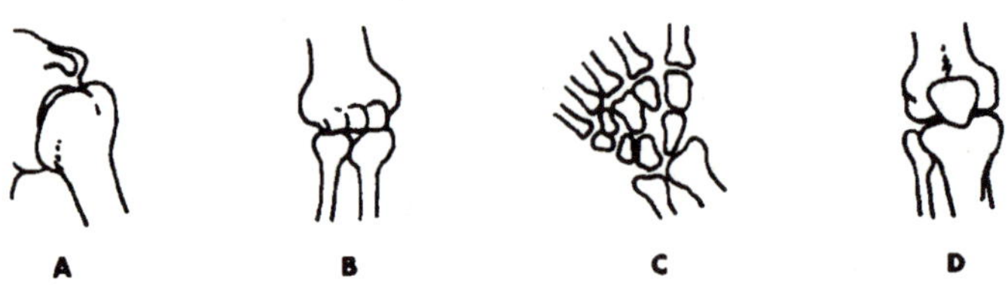

61. Refer to the illustration above. The joint shown in A is an example of a
    a. suture joint.
    b. ball-and-socket joint.
    c. pivot joint.
    d. plant joint.

    Answer: B Difficulty: II Section: 2 Objective: 5

62. Refer to the illustration above. The joint shown in D would most likely be found in the
    a. shoulder.
    b. elbow.
    c. knee.
    d. wrist.

    Answer: C Difficulty: II Section: 2 Objective: 5

63. Refer to the illustration above. Which figure shows a joint that allows bones to "glide" over each other?
    a. A
    b. B
    c. C
    d. D

    Answer: C Difficulty: II Section: 2 Objective: 5

64. Refer to the illustration above. The elbow is a hinge joint that allows your hand to turn over. It is shown in figure
    a. A.
    b. B.
    c. C.
    d. D.

    Answer: B Difficulty: II Section: 2 Objective: 5

65. Tendons connect
    a. bone to bone.
    b. muscle to bone.
    c. muscle to muscle.
    d. cartilage to bone.

    Answer: B Difficulty: I Section: 3 Objective: 1

66. A muscle can
    a. push a bone.
    b. pull a bone.
    c. both push and pull a bone simultaneously.
    d. sometimes push and sometimes pull a bone.

    Answer: B Difficulty: I Section: 3 Objective: 1

67. Muscles that function by bending joints, such as the biceps, are categorized as
    a. flexors.
    b. abductors.
    c. extensors.
    d. adductors.

    Answer: A Difficulty: I Section: 3 Objective: 1

68. Muscle cells are able to exert force by
    a. converting ADP and organic phosphate into ATP.
    b. interfering with the forces of gravity and friction.
    c. rapidly relaxing the muscle fibers.
    d. pulling on surrounding tissues.

    Answer: D Difficulty: I Section: 3 Objective: 1

69. A muscle's insertion
    a. is located on a bone that remains stationary when the muscle contracts.
    b. moves away from the origin during muscle contraction.
    c. is attached to the bone by a ligament.
    d. None of the above

    Answer: D Difficulty: I Section: 3 Objective: 1

70. The origin of a muscle
    a. is at the opposite end of the muscle from the insertion.
    b. is located on a bone that remains stationary when the muscle contracts.
    c. does not move when the muscle contracts.
    d. All of the above

    Answer: D Difficulty: I Section: 3 Objective: 1

71. flexors : bend ::
    a. immovable joints : bend
    b. slightly movable joints : be immovable
    c. extensors : straighten
    d. sutures : move a great deal

    Answer: C Difficulty: II Section: 3 Objective: 1

72. The functional unit of muscle contraction is called the
    a. myofibril.
    b. sarcomere.
    c. muscle fiber.
    d. myosin filament.

    Answer: B Difficulty: I Section: 3 Objective: 2

73. Actin and myosin
    a. are found in the sarcomeres.
    b. are proteins.
    c. interact during muscle contraction.
    d. All of the above

    Answer: D Difficulty: I Section: 3 Objective: 2

74. Repeating units of myosin and actin filaments bound by two Z lines are
    a. muscles.
    b. myofibrils.
    c. sarcomeres.
    d. extensors.

    Answer: C Difficulty: I Section: 3 Objective: 2

75. The total amount of force that a muscle can exert
    a. is determined by the strength of the nerve impulse that caused the contraction.
    b. depends on the total number of individual muscle fibers that have been stimulated.
    c. is dependent upon the weight of the object being moved.
    d. correlates to the number of Z lines contained within the sarcomeres of the muscle.

    Answer: B Difficulty: I Section: 3 Objective: 2

76. sarcomere contractions : ATP ::
    a. Z lines : actin and myosin
    b. actin and myosin : sarcomeres
    c. muscle forces : number of Z lines
    d. muscle forces : muscle fibers contracting

    Answer: D Difficulty: II Section: 3 Objective: 2

77. Aerobic activities
    a. are best for increasing muscle size and strength.
    b. produce ATP more efficiently than glycolysis.
    c. use up glycogen stores quickly.
    d. prevent myosin and actin linkages in muscles.

    Answer: B Difficulty: I Section: 3 Objective: 3

78. If you want to increase your cardiovascular endurance, the best type of exercise is
    a. anaerobic.
    b. aerobic.
    c. resistance.
    d. None of the above

    Answer: B Difficulty: I Section: 3 Objective: 3

79. If you want to increase the size and strength of your muscles, the best type of exercise is
    a. anaerobic.
    b. aerobic.
    c. resistance.
    d. None of the above

    Answer: C Difficulty: I Section: 3 Objective: 3

80. It has been known for a long time that muscle contraction requires ATP. Scientists have discovered that ATP is required to release the attachments between actin and myosin in the many cycles of attachment, release, and reattachment that result in sliding of these filaments past each other. Which of the following phenomena is explained by this specific role of ATP?
    a. muscle fatigue
    b. stiffening of a body after death (rigor mortis)
    c. opposing pairs of muscles functioning as flexors and extensors
    d. muscle sprain

    Answer: B   Difficulty: II   Section: 3   Objective: 3

81. The skin performs all of the following *except*
    a. protection.
    b. sensation of heat.
    c. control of body temperature
    d. production of gametes.

    Answer: D   Difficulty: I   Section: 4   Objective: 1

82. The thin outer layer of the skin is
    a. the dermis.
    b. the epidermis.
    c. the fatty layer.
    d. connective skin.

    Answer: B   Difficulty: I   Section: 4   Objective: 1

83. The functions of the skin include
    a. defense against microbes.
    b. regulation of body temperature.
    c. prevention of dehydration.
    d. All of the above

    Answer: D   Difficulty: I   Section: 4   Objective: 1

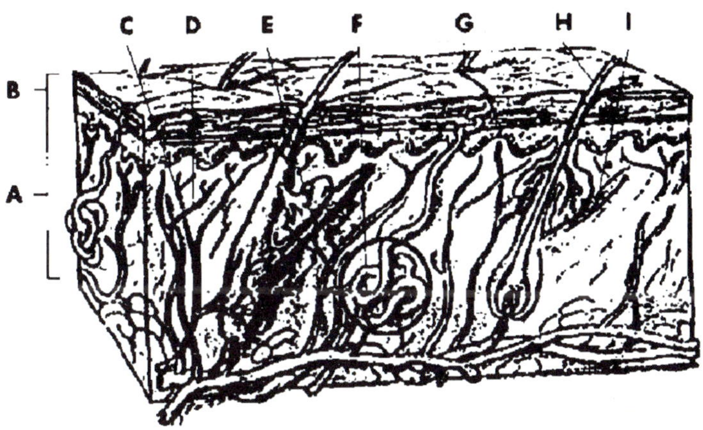

84. Refer to the illustration above. Which of the structures are composed mainly of dead cells?
    a. structures A and F
    b. structures B and H
    c. structures C and D
    d. Skin is a living organ that does not have any dead cells.

    Answer: B   Difficulty: II   Section: 4   Objective: 1

85. Refer to the illustration above. The structure labeled E
    a. often is responsible for the formation of acne.
    b. is found in adults and teenagers.
    c. may be affected by high levels of sex hormones.
    d. All of the above

    Answer: D   Difficulty: II   Section: 4   Objective: 1

86. Refer to the illustration above. Skin receives nutrients, eliminates wastes, and helps regulate body temperature by using which of the following structures?
    a. I
    b. G
    c. F
    d. D

    Answer: B   Difficulty: II   Section: 4   Objective: 2

87. Refer to the illustration above. The structure labeled F
    a. is often responsible for the formation of acne.
    b. helps regulate body temperature.
    c. is a reservoir for excess blood cells.
    d. is only found in teenagers.

    Answer: B   Difficulty: II   Section: 4   Objective: 2

88. Refer to the illustration above. The portion of the skin labeled A is
    a. the dermis.
    b. sensitive to heat and cold.
    c. composed mainly of connective tissue.
    d. All of the above

    Answer: A   Difficulty: II   Section: 4   Objective: 2

89. Keratin
    a. is a strong, fibrous protein.
    b. fills dead cells in the dermis.
    c. is a skin pigment.
    d. All of the above

    Answer: A   Difficulty: I   Section: 4   Objective: 1

90. The dermis of the skin is
    a. composed of corneal and basal layers.
    b. the innermost layer of the skin.
    c. the location of melanocytes.
    d. involved in temperature regulation.

    Answer: D   Difficulty: I   Section: 4   Objective: 2

91. Sweat glands contribute to body odor because their secretions contain
    a. carbohydrates and nucleic acids.
    b. water.
    c. proteins and fatty acids.
    d. All of the above

    Answer: C   Difficulty: I   Section: 4   Objective: 2

92. Keratin
    a. is a waterproof protein.
    b. fills dead cells in the dermis.
    c. is a skin pigment.
    d. All of the above

    Answer: A   Difficulty: I   Section: 4   Objective: 1

93. Hair and nails are produced by the cells of the
    a. dermis.
    b. subcutaneous level.
    c. subcutaneous glands.
    d. epidermis.

    Answer: D   Difficulty: I   Section: 4   Objective: 3

94. Goose bumps are caused by
    a. excessive oil production.
    b. tiny muscles in the dermis.
    c. the loss of keratin from the dermis.
    d. None of the above

    Answer: B   Difficulty: I   Section: 4   Objective: 2

95. specialized epidermal cells : nails ::
    a. "half-moon area" : hair
    b. keratin : melanocytes
    c. melanocytes : keratin
    d. hair follicles : hair

    Answer: D   Difficulty: II   Section: 4   Objective: 3

96. Overexposure to sunlight may cause all of the following *except*
    a. mutations in the skin cells.
    b. premature aging of the skin.
    c. acne.
    d. skin cancer.

    Answer: C   Difficulty: I   Section: 4   Objective: 4

97. A skin disorder caused by blockage of oil glands is called
   a. acne.
   b. carcinoma.
   c. osteoporosis.
   d. psoriasis.

   Answer: A Difficulty: I Section: 4 Objective: 4

98. The most dangerous skin cancers are called
   a. malignant keratomas.
   b. malignant melanomas.
   c. third-degree sunburn.
   d. acne.

   Answer: B Difficulty: I Section: 4 Objective: 4

99. The most effective way to reduce the risk of skin cancer includes
   a. using a sunscreen.
   b. increasing exposure to sunlight gradually.
   c. minimizing exposure to sunlight.
   d. All of the above

   Answer: C Difficulty: I Section: 4 Objective: 4

COMPLETION

100. ___________________ tissue joins, supports, and protects other types of tissue.

   Answer: Connective Difficulty: II Section: 1 Objective: 2

101. All organs of the body contain epithelial, connective, muscle, and ___________________ tissues.

   Answer: nerve Difficulty: I Section: 1 Objective: 2

102. Smooth, skeletal, and cardiac are classifications of ___________________ tissue.

   Answer: muscle Difficulty: I Section: 1 Objective: 2

103. The walls of many internal organs contain ___________________ muscle.

   Answer: smooth Difficulty: I Section: 1 Objective: 2

104. The ___________________ system is the primary organ system, which functions by breaking down food into nutrients that can be used by the body.

   Answer: digestive Difficulty: I Section: 1 Objective: 3

105. The excretory system includes the kidneys, ___________________ ___________________, ureters, and the ___________________.

   Answer: urinary bladder, urethra Difficulty: II Section: 1 Objective: 3

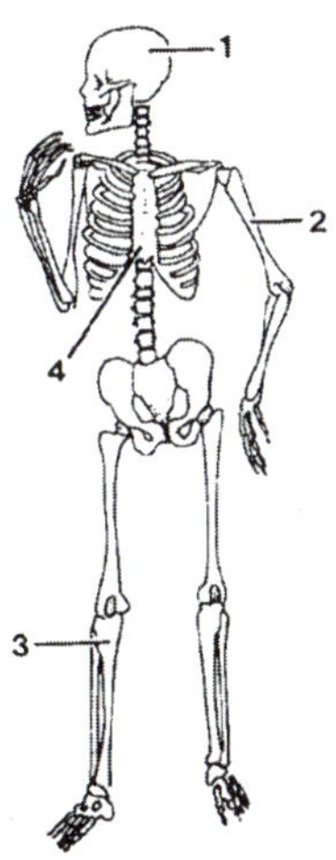

106. Refer to the illustration above. The bones labeled ___________________ and ___________________ are part of the appendicular skeleton.

   Answer: 2, 3 Difficulty: II Section: 2 Objective: 1

107. Refer to the illustration above. The bones labeled ____________________ and ____________________ are part of the axial skeleton.
Answer: 1, 4 Difficulty: II Section: 2 Objective: 1

108. The bones of the skull and backbone are part of the ____________________ skeleton.
Answer: axial Difficulty: II Section: 2 Objective: 1

109. The heart and lungs are protected by the ____________________ ____________________.
Answer: rib cage Difficulty: I Section: 2 Objective: 1

110. The bones of the arms, legs, pectoral girdle, and pelvic girdle make up the ____________________ skeleton.
Answer: appendicular Difficulty: II Section: 2 Objective: 1

111. The rib cage is formed by curved ribs extending from the backbone and joining together in the front at the bone called the ____________________.
Answer: sternum or breastbone Difficulty: I Section: 2 Objective: 1

112. The bone ____________________ inside long bones is important in blood cell production and fat storage.
Answer: marrow Difficulty: I Section: 2 Objective: 2

113. A membrane that surrounds individual bones is called the ____________________.
Answer: periosteum Difficulty: II Section: 2 Objective: 2

114. Dense, almost solid bone that provides a great deal of support is ____________________ bone.
Answer: compact Difficulty: I Section: 2 Objective: 2

115. The loss of bone density that occurs in the later years of life is known as ____________________.
Answer: osteoporosis Difficulty: I Section: 2 Objective: 4

116. The junction of two bones is called a(n) ____________________.
Answer: joint Difficulty: I Section: 2 Objective: 5

117. A painful degeneration of movable joints caused by attacks on the joints by cells of the immune system is called ____________________ ____________________.
Answer: rheumatoid arthritis Difficulty: I Section: 2 Objective: 5

118. Muscles that cause limbs to bend toward each other at a joint are called ____________________.
Answer: flexors Difficulty: II Section: 3 Objective: 1

119. Moving a bone requires the cooperation of two sets of ____________________.
Answer: muscles Difficulty: I Section: 3 Objective: 1

120. Muscles that function to straighten a joint are called ____________________.
Answer: extensors Difficulty: II Section: 3 Objective: 1

121. Strips of dense connective tissue that attach muscles to bones are called ____________________.
Answer: tendons Difficulty: I Section: 3 Objective: 1

122. Repeating units of actin and myosin filaments are called ____________________.
Answer: sarcomeres Difficulty: II Section: 3 Objective: 2

123. The most effective form of exercises to increase the size of your skeletal muscles are ____________________ exercises.
Answer: resistance Difficulty: I Section: 3 Objective: 3

124. The outermost layer of the skin is called the ________________.
Answer: epidermis Difficulty: I Section: 4 Objective: 1

125. The outer layer of the skin that contains both living and nonliving cells is called the ________________.
Answer: epidermis Difficulty: I Section: 4 Objective: 1

126. The brown pigment, ________________, is responsible for most skin color.
Answer: melanin Difficulty: I Section: 4 Objective: 1

127. Hairs grow from specialized epidermal structures called hair ________________.
Answer: follicles Difficulty: I Section: 4 Objective: 3

128. Acne is caused by overactive ________________ ________________ and hormones.
Answer: oil glands Difficulty: I Section: 4 Objective: 4

129. The most common type of skin cancers are ________________, which originate in the skin cells that do not produce pigments.
Answer: carcinomas Difficulty: II Section: 4 Objective: 4

130. Overexposure to ________________ rays may result in the mutations in skin cells that can cause skin cancer.
Answer: ultraviolet Difficulty: I Section: 4 Objective: 4

ESSAY

131. Connective tissue plays many different roles in the human body. It is crucial for providing structural support for the body. It provides protection for internal organs. It facilitates the movements of body parts. It functions in the transport of substances throughout the body. It serves a storage function for certain kinds of molecules. It also plays a vital role in enabling the body to defend itself against invading organisms or other foreign substances.

Write a short essay that first identifies the connective cell types discussed in your text. Next, distinguish these cell types from one another by their physical characteristics and by the type of matrix that is produced between the cells. Finally, relate the physical characteristics and the type of intercellular matrix to the specific function(s) that each of these cell types performs.

Answer:

Answers will vary and may include the following information:
Bone is a type of connective tissue that contains cells embedded in a matrix of collagen fibers that are coated with calcium salts. This makes bone fairly rigid and thus well-suited for providing structural support. It also provides protection of internal organs. For example, the skull protects the brain, the rib cage protects the heart and lungs, and the pelvic girdle protects organs of the reproductive, digestive, and excretory systems. Most of the human skeleton is composed of bone. Cartilage is a kind of connective tissue that contains cells embedded in a matrix of protein fibers. These fibers make cartilage strong yet flexible. Cartilage provides some structural support, particularly in young humans and at stress points between adjacent bones. Ligaments and tendons are both kinds of connective tissue that contain cells embedded in a matrix of collagen fibers. Ligaments connect bones to each other at joints, and tendons attach muscles to bones. Thus, both help the body make skeletal movements. Fibroblasts are connective tissue cells that produce collagen and secrete it. This collagen is then used as the intercellular matrix of the other types of connective tissue that contain collagen. Blood is a kind of connective tissue that contains cells embedded in a matrix of water. Blood is the medium in which oxygen, nutrients, wastes, hormones, antibodies, and many other chemicals are transported to and from the cells of the body. Some of the blood cells function as part of the immune system, and other cells defend our bodies against

invading organisms and foreign substances. Some of these cells, such as macrophages, ingest and destroy any such harmful agent. Other cells, such as lymphocytes, are involved in attacks against specific harmful agents. Adipose tissue is a kind of connective tissue that contains cells embedded in a matrix of mostly collagen fibers. The cells store fat as an energy reserve for our bodies.

Difficulty: III Section: 1 Objective: 2

132. Give an example of each of the following types of tissue, and briefly describe its functions: epithelial tissue, muscle tissue, connective tissue, and nerve tissue.

Answer:

Epithelial tissues, such as skin, are generally flat sheets of cells that protect the body from damage and control water loss in the tissues that they cover. Muscle tissue moves the body structures (skeletal muscle) and moves materials through the body (cardiac and smooth muscle). Connective tissue defends the body from invaders (white blood cells), sequesters materials (fat, melanin), and supports the body (bone and cartilage). Nerve tissues (brain, spinal cord) carry information in the form of electrical impulses throughout the body.

Difficulty: III Section: 1 Objective: 2

133. List the three types of muscle tissue, and give the function of each.

Answer:

The three types of muscle tissue are skeletal muscle, cardiac muscle, and smooth muscle. Skeletal muscle moves bones, and cardiac muscle pumps blood through the body. Smooth muscle moves food through the body and performs other internal functions including changing blood vessel diameter, opening and closing bronchioles, and causing uterine contractions during labor.

Difficulty: III Section: 1 Objective: 2

134. How does maintaining a relatively warm body temperature (endothermy) help humans?

Answer:

Endothermy permits the body to maintain its activity at all times and in many different places, regardless of the temperature of the surroundings. In addition, endothermy allows the body to sustain strenuous activity. Ectotherms, by contrast, are limited to short periods of exertion.

Difficulty: III Section: 1 Objective: 4

135. Why is it essential for the body to maintain homeostasis?

Answer:

A stable fluid environment is necessary for multicellular organisms. Any extreme change in extracellular fluid can have very serious effects on the activities inside cells. If factors such as pH level, ion concentration, and sugar level vary outside the range that cells require, death may result.

Difficulty: III Section: 1 Objective: 4

136. List five types of freely movable joints in your body, and give a location for each.

Answer:

Ball-and-socket joints are found in the shoulders and hip. Pivot joints enable heads to rotate and are found at the top of spines. Gliding joints are found in wrists and ankles. Saddle joints function at the base of thumbs. The knees, elbows, and knuckles provide examples of hinge joints.

Difficulty: III Section: 2 Objective: 5

137. Using examples, describe the three basic types of joints and their primary functions.

Answer:

Immovable joints are very tight joints that hold adjacent bones together, permitting little or no movement. The cranial bones of the skull are held together by virtually immovable joints called sutures. Limited mobility is permitted by slightly movable joints, the second basic type of joint. In these joints, a bridge of cartilage joins two bones together, as in the joints between the vertebrae of the spine. The third type of joint is the freely movable joint. These joints allow the greatest degree of movement. They are found between bones that are held together by ligaments.

Difficulty: III Section: 2 Objective: 5

138. What is a ligament? What does it mean if a ligament is sprained? Explain.

Answer:

A ligament is a tough connective tissue that joins one bone to another. Although ligaments are very elastic, there is a limit to how far they can stretch. When a ligament is stretched too far, the injury that results is called a sprain.

Difficulty: III Section: 2 Objective: 5

139. Describe the contraction of muscle according to the sliding filament theory.

Answer:

Myosin and actin filaments lie in parallel lines along the length of a myofibril in units called sarcomeres. The myosin heads touch the adjacent actin filaments. When a muscle contracts, the myosin heads attach to the actin filaments, and when the heads bend inward, they pull the actin filaments along with them, toward each other. As the actin filaments move toward each other along the myosin filament, they pull their Z lines with them, thus shortening the sarcomere. As sarcomeres are shortened along the entire muscle fiber, the entire muscle contracts. ATP is used as the myosin head detaches from the binding site and snaps back into its original position.

Difficulty: III Section: 3 Objective: 2

140. The skin is composed of three layers. What are they, and what do they do?

Answer:

The outermost layer of the skin is the epidermis. This layer is responsible for protection from the environment. The epidermis produces new cells from its deepest layer (the basal layer) that move upward to become the corneal layer. Accessory structures, such as hair and nails, are produced by cells of the epidermis. The middle and thickest layer of the skin is called the dermis, which is the major framework of the skin. This layer provides structural support and is a matrix for nerve endings, blood vessels, and the specialized cells of the skin. The subcutaneous layer is the innermost layer of the skin. This is a layer of fat-rich cells that act as shock absorbers, provide insulation, and store vitamins.

Difficulty: III Section: 4 Objective: 1

141. How does the skin help regulate body temperature?

Answer:

Nerves in the skin sense heat, providing stimuli that dilate or constrict blood vessels. When the temperature in the environment is high, blood vessels dilate, allowing body heat to escape. Also, the skin produces sweat through its sweat glands, and the evaporation of sweat has a cooling effect on the body. When the temperature of the environment is low, blood vessels in the skin contract, reducing heat loss.

Difficulty: III Section: 4 Objective: 2

142. What are three functions of the blood vessels in the dermis? Describe each function.

Answer:

The blood vessels in the dermis provide nutrient-rich blood to nourish skin cells, to carry away cellular waste products, and to regulate body temperature. Blood radiates heat into the air as it passes near the surface of the skin. If the body becomes too hot, these blood vessels enlarge, allowing more blood to flow through the dermis near the body surface.

Difficulty: III Section: 4 Objective: 2

143. What causes acne? Can it be prevented or controlled?

Answer:

Acne is caused by several factors including hormones and an increase in oil production by glands during adolescence. Excessive oil production can clog the oil glands, causing a buildup of oil, dirt, and bacteria. While acne cannot be prevented, the conditions associated with it may be controlled with proper skin care.

Difficulty: III Section: 4 Objective: 4

9997266153 1 2 3 4 5 6